CERTIFIED NURSE ASSISTANT'S EXAM QUESTIONS AND ANSWERS FOR LONG TERM CARE CERTIFICATION

STUDY GUIDE

Daphna Moore LMT CMT NA

Many Questions and Answers Given on All State Board CNA Exams

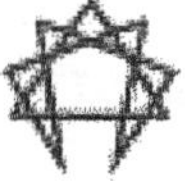

Hughes Henshaw Publications LLC
Palm Bay, FL 342907

JANUARY 2009

CERTIFIED NURSE ASSISTANTS EXAM QUESTIONS FOR LONG TERM CARE CERTIFICATION STUDY GUIDE

Library of Congress Cataloging in Publication Data

Moore, Daphna

Certified nurse assistant's exam questions for long term care certification

INTERNATIONAL STANDARD BOOK NUMBER:

ISBN 978-1-892693-42-6

1. Nursing — Examinations, questions, etc. 2. Nuses' aides-Examinations — Study Guides. I. Title.

RT84.M66 1999
610.73'076–dc21

99-12413

CIP

HUGHES HENSHAW PUBLICATIONS LLC
PALM BAY, FL 32907

(321) 956-8885 Office
(321) 956-2475 Fax
www.hugheshenhsaw.com

ABOUT THE AUTHOR

Daphna Moore, studied and passed her Nurse Assisting at the largest Long Term Care Facility in Denver, CO, and became a Nurse Assistant upon completion of her final exam. She also taught Massage Therapy and was a practicing Massage Therapist for over 20 years in Colorado.

In 1976 she attended Lotus Lodge, a Wholistic Retreat in Strasburg, OH, taking various modalities: massage, iridology, nutrition, color therapy, etc. In the summer of 1979 and 1980 she attended classes at the Healing Light Center in Glendale, CA with Roslyn Bruyer and studied Aura Balancing, energy modalities, etc. In 1980 and 1981 she took a 6-month class on Touch for Health Textbook by John F. Thie, D.C. in Boulder, CO. This included muscle testing, meridians and oriental philosophy. She became a member of the AMTA in February 1986, (graduated under a previous married name) and continued her studies and created various tests for students in order to help them pass massage certification exams.

In 1989 and 1990 she attended a few workshops at the Colorado School of Traditional Chinese Medicine in Denver, CO. These classes were for gaining knowledge and not for any credit toward a degree. She also studied ANMA, the art of Japanese Massage, in Boulder, CO, not for credit but for additional knowledge. During the early 80's she took classes in hypnosis in Denver, CO, and became a hypno-therapist in 1981 utilizing this for past life regressions. She also became a Nurse Assistant in the mid 80's.

TABLE OF CONTENTS

CHAPTER ONE
Ideas and Insights From Wise CNAs

This Chapter covers what they had to say at the CNA Leadership Conferences.

ON THE SURVEY PROCESS...

How can the CNA help in the survey process?

- Don't panic!
- Practice good hand washing
- See that the residents have privacy
- Attend to repositioning
- Participate in activities, offer fluids, help at meals, and don't just walk by residents
- Respond to behavioral problems:
  - redirect
  - get help
  - know in advance what's to be done

COMMENT: ***I'm so sick of the games they (supervisory staff) play during survey. Administrative staff comes out on the floor and pretend they work like that all the time.***

ON CARE GIVING TO RESIDENTS...

I'm lead tech. I really enjoy the people (at my facility). I do scheduling, so I don't just walk away after I post my schedules. I make sure people are being changed. CNAs will come to me and say, "This resident won't take a bath." I calm the resident down, let them know I care, and am trying to help.

I remember that residents are human beings, even though they are in a nursing home; so I treat them with respect and dignity. I know I really do make a big difference in their lives by enhancing residents' rights. I hate to miss a day of work knowing they will miss my help.

When a resident doesn't want to be bathed, I just ask the resident to go for a walk with me - to the shower room without letting them know why. Then when I get them in there, I explain to them why we're in there. It is only after they refuse me in the shower room that I accept their refusal.

I really don't try to trick residents. I just try to keep a smile on my face and be myself. It takes more muscles to frown than to smile.

I give residents choices of what they would like to wear. I notify them in advance of bathing and of meals. I ask if they want a nap or not. Just plain give them a choice. If you hand them a wash cloth, they will wash their own face.

ON DEALING WITH DEMENTIA AND DIFFICULT BEHAVIORS...

- Set limits with behavior validation therapy; protect others from behaviors.
- Deal with the patient's depression.
- Each patient is an individual and needs different approaches.
- Enter the resident's world of reality. Behaviors occur when you try to bring them to our reality. Residents still want to control their lives. Allow them that control.

When a resident is wandering and trying every door to the outside, sometimes some people want to put that resident in the locked unit; but if the resident can just be taken outside for five minutes, the wandering and trying to get out usually dissipates.

Staff often tries to reason or argue with one of our residents who is very argumentative by nature. This only agitates her. One CNA de-escalates the situation by acting funny / crazy, which causes the resident to laugh and relax. The resident likes the aid and feels that the aid understands her and is a real friend.

A resident refused to get up. She got mad at the aid, who wanted to help her get up. The resident stayed mad throughout the shift and stayed in bed. The aid worked a second shift and continued to visit the resident, filling ice water and other little things. Then she apologized for offending the resident by wanting to assist her in the morning. The resident apologized to the aid. Now the aid and the resident are best buddies.

We had an Alzheimer's resident who was hesitant and resistant to walking any distance. The restorative aid encouraged the resident to wave at others while walking a few feet each day. The aid continued to increase the distance. The resident waved each day on her walks. It took three months to reach the end of the hall. At last, the resident could say "hi" to all her new friends she had been waving at daily.

When a resident is combative:

- Redirect or leave for five minutes and try again.
- Try to redirect, find a common topic to talk about to direct him/her.
- We need to watch our body language!

When a resident rummages through other people's things:

- Provide a drawer to rummage through.
- Suggest to the resident that someone must have borrowed the item she is looking for but they'll bring it back.

When a resident is sexually inappropriate:

- Use firm words, ("Please remove your hand").
- If in private and not involving or offending others, just leave the resident alone.

Getting a resident to bath when they refuse:

- Try again in a while and be persistent.
- Use yourself as the one who needs help in getting the job done.
- Use incentives (ice cream helps).
- Talk with the resident; be gentle.
- If a resident is real stubborn sponge or bed baths are okay.
- Talk to the family for information and tips; perhaps they might know a better approach.
- Be alert to old rituals or routines.
- Residents feel CNAs are in a hurry. Make them feel unrushed.

Dealing with families:

- Nursing homes are viewed as warehouses.
- Reassure families.
- Sometimes families are harder to deal with than residents.
- Make only promises you can keep to families and residents.

CHAPTER TWO

What the CNAs Had To Say About the Work of CNAs At the CNA Leadership Conferences

WHAT DO YOU NEED TO BE HAPPIER IN YOUR WORK?

- **$$$$** I've been in this work for a long time. My income is still too low to qualify for a credit card.
- Pay - Better raises and benefits.
- Pay increase. If facilities offered me what they paid pool staff, I would work extra shifts. Money is always a great incentive, especially if you're working short staffed and are really stressed out.
- Pool staff gets two times what regular CNAs make. They arrive late but still get paid for a full shift.
- Pay extra for child care.
- Fully staffed facility; bonus incentives; cheap child care.
- We need some kind of procedures to teach teamwork.
- I've been working in this for a few years now. What we need is team work. Where I work they don't give bonuses or even say thank you.

    - ***My Christmas bonus was a $5 gift card to Block Buster Video. I hadn't worked a full year yet (so that's all I got.)***
    - ***(Response from a different facility): After one year we got a $65 Christmas bonus and it goes up every year. You'd think they'd want to show some appreciation of the new employees too.***

- More incentives would be free meals and bonus money.
- Higher beginning wage for a nursing home CNA since the level of work is much harder.

- A good benefit would be tuition reimbursement for going to school.
- Make scholarships available.
- More residents means more paper work; more residents with fewer CNAs means more work per person to do and stress levels are raised.
- Staff develops bad attitudes when they are always called in at the last minute - limits personal life.
- Create a range of pay scales, on levels, such as 1-4, etc. for CNAs, according to their skills.
- The CNA population has changed. Aids are younger. Training needs to change to fit the needs of younger trainees.

REGARDING NURSES:

CO-WORKERS COMMENT: ***A role model for me is a nurse, Roni, who will answer a call light. I'm not used to that. Roni is a model to me, too. She does staffing but also runs around and helps.***

- We need more training for nurses
- Educate nurses and other personnel to appreciate CNAs.
- Some charge nurses treat us worse than the residents do.
- One nurse says we're being disrespectful if the CNAs offer their observations about care. Then she doesn't pass along what we've told her and blames ***us (the CNAs)*** if resident's needs are not identified.
- There's a difference between bitchy and strict. Strick is OK if she lets you do your job.

- CNAs aren't all treated equal. The nurses have favorites.
- If we try to talk to someone over the charge nurse's head, it comes back to us. It's not worth it.
- Administration gives everything to the nurses and nothing to the CNAs. Some workers and some CNAs have worked there for ***many*** years, and they have gotten ***NO*** bonuses.
- Nurses who don't participate in care, don't listen, don't answer calls, etc. cause a lot of problems.

COMMENT: ***A bell is ringing in a room. It seems the only time they will ever answer it is when the state authorities are there. Why is this? This causes problems also.***

SELF ESTEEM AND PROFESSIONALISM...

What can YOU do to improve the reality of your work environment?

- CNAs need to work and treat each other as human beings. Nurses too! Never ask anyone to do something that you wouldn't do. By doing this you can give love to each other and to the residents.
- Go back to school to become an RN. Then the benefits would be sick days, retirement, and health insurance.
- Love the work you are doing with your peers and for the residents.
- Work together - helping everyday with the most you can do
- Be a good team player. Communicate!
- Respect EVERYONE in the work you do.
- Improve the quality of care to all the residents.
- Acknowledge reality - see the big picture - and try to do something about it.

- Communicate better with other departments (dietary, PT, etc.).
- Joke and have fun with your co-workers.
- (At our facility) we really do well as a team. We listen to each other and communicate really well. Each floor has a nurse manager who's there for us to talk to about our problems.
- Residents will feel it if our self-esteem is poor. We need to keep ourselves ***up*** so they'll be ***up.***
- A positive attitude will produce positive results. Then work is not drudgery or a task; it's natural.
- Don't be a *"no-call, no-show."* You cheat your own self by doing so.
- Swap shifts if you need to so in order not to miss work.
- I don't think of my job as a *paycheck*. It comes from my heart. If it doesn't come from your heart, then you should go somewhere where you are more satisfied in what you are doing.
- Take care of these people like you want to be taken care of.
- Don't do too many doubles. I fill in by coming in early, but not always a whole shift. I have to take care of myself first, or I will be no good to the residents.

Practical tips for co-workers

- My daily goal is to reach somebody in a positive way, regardless of what I'm doing. Try to be *up.*
- Try to find the positive in every situation.
- Attitude ripples out to others.
- We're bonded to each other so we can look to each other and fall back on each other.

What are some other things that enhance self esteem?

- It's a reward when a resident calls you by your name or smiles at you.
- The residents and family members give us our self-esteem
- We'll always be needed. You can't get a computer to do peri-care!
- The rewards surpass the *bad* stuff.

After a weekend off, the residents tell you they missed you.
Self-esteem builds more when people notice the work you do.

Components of Professionalism:

- attendance
- appearance
- the way you present yourself, including language
- respect for one other
- positive conduct
- increase your knowledge
- good personality
- good sense of humor
- achievement (by doing your very best)
- work hard
- stay focused on what you are doing
- be sensitive
- good P.R.(Public Relations)
- maintain a good attitude
- be proud of your accomplishments

How can the administration help you?

- Working side by side with us and understanding what we do all day.

- Talking with all of the CNAs about care concerns.
- The Administration needs to understand truly the workload and the stress of a CNA, and how many bosses we really have. Also have department heads assist in different departments when we're short of help.
- Have peer group meetings and meetings with administration where CNAs could voice their needs and their concerns regarding working conditions.
- We need ***caring administrators***. When they ask us, "How are your doing?", they should mean it. We should be able to be honest when asked about things, and maybe get a little help with resident care, when we are so rushed.
- ***I think that everyone in administration should be CNA certified. Then they would understand the concept of teamwork.***
- All staff should have social skills training.
- We do lots of staff pot-lucks including housekeeping and kitchen work, not just nursing. It brings us closer. Evening shifts should have pot-lucks, also.

> **COMMENT:** ***A key is when the administrative staff supports the workers. Our administrator, Mr. ------, makes rounds. He makes himself known and visible to staff and residents. My last administrator only came out when he was*** **in a tirade...*****They always tell us how good we are. Mr. _____ always pats us on the back. We all pitch in - we're like at home. We bitch and fight like some families but we're always there for each other!***

Why do you think you have not been able to change administration to give you more help?

- We, as a team, do not know how to approach the problem.
- I think that some CNAs can't talk about things to administrators.

- Even though they say CNAs are the backbone of the facility, they don't really believe it.
- Administration is so busy they don't think about the fact that the bell is ringing, the puddle is on the floor. They are capable of answering the bell to at least find out whether a CNA is needed or not. They are capable of mopping up the puddle if everyone is rushing around.
- We have brought things up to Administrations attention and we were told that it would be talked about. ***That's the last we ever hear of it.***
- Too many closed doors. "I'm busy, go talk with Mr. Smith." And the chain continues.
    - *Like it or not, we are looked down on in our field. We're the cleaner-uppers. People say, "How can you do that job?"*
    - *The government has forgotten how important the CNAs are. We are put aside.*

What is the most difficult problems with your co-workers?

- Some do not want to do team work - just do their own work.
- When you help them, they say THEY did it, and then they don't even say thank you.
- Trying to get them to adapt to new ideas and systems. Also getting them to understand the importance of teamwork.
- Co-workers wanting to do their own job first
- Some don't care. It's hard to be the one who does all the caring and therefore most of the work.
- Not spending any time with the patients after they get them up. Not checking on them to see if they need anything.
- It's everyone's responsibility to understand everyone needs to pitch in.

IMPROVING COMMUNICATION:

- Have administration walk a mile in my shoes.
- Have a communication book for all departments.
- Staff development should know the job descriptions for everyone in their facility.
- If there's been a misunderstanding with a co-worker, approach the person involved either by writing a note or talking with them.

SUGGESTIONS FOR RESTORATIVE NURSING

- Have regular CNAs fill in for restorative CNAs
- More training on restorative in CNA classes
- Need more restorative staff and more education for restorative aids.

CARING FOR THE CARE GIVER - CARING FOR YOURSELF

If the goal is to stay sane and healthy while doing your best - how do you accomplish this?

> ***Whether its work support or moral support, we get it from one another. Sometimes we trade off to get a break regarding a particularly difficult resident. We really feel like we're family and we take care of each other.***

- know your own strengths and weaknesses
- don't mix work and family
- take mental and emotional breaks
- good teamwork, good attitude
- you don't have to respond to every wish of every resident
- know the difference between what people want and what they really need

- start the day with a good attitude - if you start tense, the whole day will be tense
- meditate - keep quiet and breathe - even if you have to go in the bathroom and shut the door for five minutes - find calm
- pray a little and even sing to yourself sometime
- think of a peaceful place - for some it could be the ocean, forest, or mountain streams
- condition our emotions by taking a few minutes to find peace and calm
- finish every day and be done with it
- don't take your work home with you, physically or mentally
- once a week have breakfast in bed, even if you have to fix it yourself
- listen to music in the car between patients (home-health aid)
- if you're good at geriatrics, then you need to serve them (the elderly); and know you can do it as it is a very special gift. **Love the residents!**

The CNA Bill of Rights

Developed By the Participants of the 1998 CNA Leadership Conference

1. The right to be treated with consideration and respect.
2. The right to be fairly compensated.
3. The right to good training and supervision
4. The right to voice a grievance without fear of reprisal
5. The right to be appreciated and understood.
6. The right to be treated as an adult.
7. The right to have support when residents become abusive
8. The right to voice our own opinions.
9. The right to adequate staffing
10. The right to a safe work environment
11. The right to adequate equipment and supplies.
12. The right to receive positive feedback.
13. The right to privacy.
14. The right to have a private place for breaks and meals
15. The right to access public telephone
16. The right to have more than one bathroom
17. The right to be informed of infectious diseases.
18. The right to attend high quality assurance meetings.
19. The right to pick up a paycheck without attending a meeting.
20. The right to a reasonable workload for an 8 hour shift.
21. The right to be included in resident care plans.
22. The right to receive a status report before each shift.
23. The right not to be judged for our personal beliefs.
24. The right to know if there is a complaint about us.
25. The right for follow-up on a grievance.
26. The right to use the chain of command if a complaint goes unresolved.
27. The right to be reprimanded in private.
28. The right to be treated like a professional.

29. The right not to be intimidated by administration.
30. The right to leave in the event of a personal emergency.
31. The right to refuse to do a procedure that we have not been trained on.
32. The right to be called by my name.
33. The right to a comfortable work environment.
34. The right to be a valued member of the team.
35. The right to advance in our position.
36. The right to have advocates for CNAs.

CHAPTER THREE
Tasks Allowed for CNA Skilled
Tasks NOT Allowed for PCP Non-Skilled

TASK	CNA / SKILLED ** (not allowed for PCP)	PCP NON-SKILLED (allowed for PCP)
Ambulation- Assist: crutch, walker, cane, wheelchair, braces*	Considered skilled when: skilled transfers are required with the ambulation; pt. is still being trained in the use of adaptive equipment; there is the need for observation and reporting to the nurse when assisting someone in a new cast; or there is the need for skilled skin care (see skin care)	Non-skilled when: client is fully trained with adaptive equipment; no skilled transfer is required; no need for observation or reporting to the nurse for someone with a cast; or no need for skilled skin care. Adaptive equipment may include, but is not limited to gait belts/ walkers/canes/ wheelchairs.
Use of Warm and Cool Applications	Task would fall under expanded role or delegation with appropriate nursing oversight.	
BATH: Bed, tub, shower; Back rub; Skin care*	A bath is skilled when skilled skin care, skilled transfer or skilled dressing is required. SKIN CARE is skilled when there is broken skin, or potential for infection due to a chronic skin-condition in an active state. Skin care includes wound care, dressing changes, delegated application of prescription medications (ie: lotions etc.), skilled observation and reporting, but does not include use of sterile technique.	Bathing is non-skilled when no skilled skin care, dressing or transfer is required. SKIN CARE is non-skilled only when the skin is not broken and there is no active chronic skin problem. Non-skilled care must be of preventive rather than a therapeutic nature, it may include application of non-medicated or over the counter lotions and solutions. Also, non-skilled skin care would be the rubbing of reddened areas, reporting of changes to supervisor and the application of preventive spray on unbroken skin areas that may be susceptible to development of decubiti.

TASK	CNA/SKILLED (not allowed for PCP)	PCP NON-SKILLED (allowed for PCP)
Positioning of the Patient	POSITIONING may include simple alignment in a bed, wheelchair, or other furniture. POSITIONING is considered skilled when the pt. is not able to identify to the care giver when the position needs to be changed, and when skilled skin care is needed in conjunction with the positioning. The presence of communicable disease, therapeutic beds, (Clinitron, Stryker, Circle), casts or traction equipment, draining wounds, an unconscious or dying patient would require additional instruction and nursing over site.	POSITIONING is considered non-skilled only when the client is able to identify to the care giver when the position needs to be changed, and only when skilled skin care is not required in conjunction with the positioning.

CONTINUE FOR
BOWEL AND BLADDER
ELIMINATION

TASK	CNA/SKILLED (not allowed for PCP)	PCP NON-SKILLED (allowed for PCP
BOWEL & BLADDER Elimination: Bed pan/urinal; care of the incontinent pt.; Stoma care (colostomy, ileostomy) Bowel/Bladder training; Maintenance programs including CATHETER CARE: empty bag, cleanse tubing and bag, perineal care, external catheter care.*	BLADDER Care is skilled when it involves disruption of the closed system for a oley or suprapubic catheter, such as changing from a leg bag to a night bag. Care of external catheters is also considered skilled. BOWEL CARE is considered skilled when skilled transfer or skilled skin care is required in conjunction with the bowel care. Skilled bowel care includes: bowel programs with digital stimulation and enemas; care of ostomies that are new; and care of ostomies when the client is unable to self-direct the care, provided that sterile technique is not required. SKILLED CARE may include: irrigation of established colostomies and ileostomies; care of neurogenic bowel/bladder; patients with open skin/wounds, decubiti, stomas, burns, casts, requiring specific nursing oversight	BLADDER CARE is considered non-skilled only when there is no skilled transfer, or skilled skin care involved in conjunction with the bladder care. Non-skilled care may include: assisting the client to and from the bathroom; assistance with bed pans, urinals, and commodes; and changing of clothing and/or pads used for the care of incontinence. Emptying of foley bags is considered non-skilled only if there is no disruption of the closed system; the PCP must be trained to understand what constitutes disruption of the closed system. BOWEL CARE is considered non-skilled when: there is no skilled transfer or skin care in conjunction with the bowel care(i.e. Assistance to and from the bathroom, use of bed pans, and/or commodes.) The changing of clothing and/or pads of any kind for the care of incontinence is considered non-skilled. Emptying of ostomy bags and assistance with other client-directed ostomy care is non-skilled only when there is no need for reporting of observations to a nurse.
Care of Convulsive Patient; Recognition of levels of consciousness and protection of the patient, obtaining assistance.	Documentation of seizure activity, protection etc., would fall under an expanded role or delegation with appropriate nursing oversight.	
Decubitus; prevention care	Care is skilled when there is broken skin, special therapeutic regimen, or draining wounds (also see skin care).	

TASK	CNA/SKILLED (Not allowed for PCP)	PCP NON-SKILLED (allowed for PCP)
Care of the diabetic patient; use ofdipsticks, glucometers, or other automatic lancets; recognize hypo or hyperglycemic systems.	Care is skilled when the task falls under expanded role or delegation with appropriate nursing oversight. This could include capillary blood collection if supervised by a competent patient, or assisting a patient in positioning an automatic lancet. Actual finger sticks are not within the CNA scope of practice, they can only be delegated by the RN.	
Dressing:- assist with getting dressed.	Dressing is considered skilled when skilled skin care or transfer is required in conjunction with the dressing. The application of antiembolic or other pressure stockings obtained with a physician's prescription is considered skilled. Application of orthopedic devices such as splints, braces, and artificial limbs; if considerable manipulation of the device or limb is necessary, or if the patient is learning to use, the device or limb at the direction of a therapist or appropriate professional is considered skilled.	Dressing is considered non-skilled when no skilled skin care or transfers are involved. Non-skilled dressing may include assistance with ordinary clothing, application of support stockings of the type non requiring a physician's order, application of orthopedic devices such as splints, braces, or artificial limbs, if considerable manipulation of the device is not necessary, and the patient is fully trained in the use of the device.
Dressings - apply: clean technique, simple dressings, binders, ace bandages, support stockings	Task would fall under expanded role or delegation with appropriate nursing oversight. (Also see skin care, and decubitus care)	
Care of the dying patient	Physical care as directed by the Hospice or HHA nurse, including emotional support	Emotional support may be provided if the pt is covered by HCBS/PCP services as well as Hospice or HHA services.

TASK	CNA / SKILLED (not allowed for PCP)	PCP NON-SKILLED (allowed for PCP)
Enemas Intake/Output	Skilled care under the direction of the nurse (see BOWEL care) task may fall under expanded role or delegation when appropriate and might include checking for impaction, measuring fluid intake/output etc.	
Exercises and Positioning: Passive range of motion	Assistance with exercised is considered skilled when the exercises are prescribed by a nurse or other licensed medical professional. This may include passive range of motion, or working with simple traction, fractures, casts, dislocation, paralysis, contracture, unconscious, or technology depend patients.	Assistance with exercises is non-skilled when the exercises are not prescribed by a nurse or health professional. Non-skilled assistance is limited to the encouragement of normal bodily movement, as tolerated by the client.
Fluids and Nourishment: preparation, menu planning, encouraging fluids	Providing nourishment or feeding is considered skilled when skilled skin care or skilled dressing (ie. Due to presence of tracheostomy, fistulas, the inability of the patient to sit, difficulty in swallowing, or infants and/or children) is required in conjunction with the feeding and when oral suctioning is needed on a stand-by or other basis. This includes syringe feeding. Skilled feeding requires prior nursing assessment of the patient before the expanded role is assigned.	Feeding is non-skilled when skin care or dressing is not required (as described under CNA Skilled), in conjunction with the feeding and when oral suctioning is not needed on any basis. Non-skilled feeding includes assistance with eating by mouth, using common eating utensils, such as forms, knives, and spoons.
Hair Care: shampoo bed shampoo	Hair care is skilled when performed in conjunction with skilled skin care, transfer, or dressing as described previously. Care is skilled in the presence of traction, hair loss from radiation, drugs, psoriasis, pediculosis, or other infection.	Hair care is non-skilled when there is no skilled skin, transfer, or dressing care involved. Hair care under these limitations may include shampooing with non-medicated shampoo or shampoo that doesn't require a physician's order, drying, styling, or combing of hair.

TASK	CNA / SKILLED (not allowed for PCP)	PCP NON-SKILLED (allowed for PCP)
Medications	Medication ASSISTANCE is considered skilled care, and consists of putting the medication in the client's hand/mouth when the patient is physically unable but can self-direct the taking of the medication	Medication REMINDING is allowed as unskilled personal care **ONLY** when medications have been preselected by the client, a family member, a nurse, or a pharmacist, and are stored in containers other than prescription bottles, i.e. such as medication minders. Medication minder containers must be clearly marked as to day and time of dosage, and must be kept in such a way as to prevent tampering. Medication reminding includes only inquiries as to whether medications were taken, verbal prompting to take medications, handing the appropriately marked med minder container to the client, and opening the appropriately marked med minder compartment when the client is physically unable. Medication reminding does **NOT** include taking the medication out of the container. These limitations apply to all prescription and OTC medications including PRN medications. Any irregularities noted in the preselected medications, such as meds taken too often, or not often enough, not taken at the correct time as marked on the med minder, shall be reported to the supervisor immediately.
Nail Care	Nail care (fingers and toes) is skilled when skilled skin care is required in conjunction with the nail care, and in the presence of medical conditions that may involve peripheral circulatory problems or loss of sensation. This includes cleaning, filing, trimming with clippers.	Nail care is considered non-skilled when no skilled skin care is involved in conjunction with the nail care, and only in the absence of any medical conditions that might involve peripheral circulatory problems or loss of sensation. Nail care under these limitations may include soaking of the nails, pushing back cuticles, and trimming and filing of nails.

TASK	CNA / skilled (not allowed for PCP)	PCP NON-SKILLED (allowed for PCP)
Observation, reporting and documentation	Skilled care is the documenting of services/tasks provided according to the assignment sheet developed by the RN. Includes the recognition and reporting of emergencies, as well as variations from established parameters requiring further assessment and/or intervention from the nurse.	Non-skilled documentation is the checking off of the tasks/services provided to the client under the direction of the supervisor.
Personal Hygiene; oral hygiene, and dental care	Per assessment and assignment by the RN oral/mouth care is considered skilled when: skilled skin care is required in conjunction with the mouth care; when there is injury or disease of the face, mouth, head or neck; in the presence of communicable disease; when the patient is unconscious; or when oral suctioning is required.	Mouth/oral care is considered non-skilled ONLY when skilled skin care is not required in conjunction with the oral care. Mouth care under these limitations may include denture care and basic oral hygiene.
Respiratory	Respiratory care is skilled care, and includes postural drainage, cupping, adjusting oxygen flow within established parameters, and suctioning of mouth and nose. Skilled care may involve reinforcement of safety precautions, and cleaning of equipment and tubing.	Respiratory care is considered skilled. However, PCPs may clean the tubing for oxygen equipment and may temporarily remove and replace the cannula or mask from the client's face for purposes of shaving or washing the client's face. Adjustments to the oxygen flow are NOT allowed.
Shaving	Shaving is skilled when performed in conjunction with skilled skin care; an electric razor or safety razor may be used, depending on the medical condition.	Shaving is considered non-skilled only when skilled skin care is not involved, and ONLY an electric razor may be used.
Specimen collection	As assigned by the nurse, the CNA may assist with the collection of urine, stool, or sputum samples.	

TASK	CNA / SKILLED (not allowed for PCP)	PCP NON-SKILLED (Allowed for PCP)
Transfers: weight bearing, non-weight bearing	Assistance with transfers is considered skilled when the client is unable to assist with the transfer. Use of Hoyer lifts is considered skilled, and use of other adaptive equipment is considered skilled if the patient is still being trained in the use of the equipment.	Assistance with transfers is considered unskilled only when the client has sufficient balance and strength to assist with the transfer to some extent. Except for Hoyer lifts, adaptive equipment may be used in transfers, provided the client is fully trained in the use of the equipment and can direct the transfer. Adaptive equipment may include, but is not limited to , gait belts, wheelchairs, tub seats and grab bars.
Take and record VITAL SIGNS: TPR / BP, weight and record	Taking of vital signs is considered skilled. The RN will set parameters for each patient as necessary, and the CNA will notify the RN when readings are outside of the set parameters.	
Maintains clean, safe and healthy environment including infection control procedures	As necessary to meet the needs of the patient, the CNA will clean the area specific to the patient, (this is incidental to the skilled aide services provided). The CNA will be trained in universal precautions as required to care for the patient.	Non-skilled care is limited to routine house cleaning.
Oriented to and understands: Patient's Rights, and Confidential issues	Included in agency orientation	Included in agency orientation.

TASK	CNA / SKILLED (not allowed for PCP)	PCP NON-SKILLED (allowed for PCP)
Communication skills	Skilled communication skills require the CNA o be able to document in the record, observations and services delivered as the extension of the nurse. See observation reporting and documenting.	See observation, reporting, and documenting
Transport of patients and the providing of financial management		PCPs shall not transport clients, however PCPs may accompany the client to medical appointments and to other services as specified on the care plan when all the care that is provided by the PCP in relation to the trip is non-skilled. PCPs shall not provide financial management.
Protective Oversight		Protective oversight is considered non-skilled when the client requires standby assistance with any of the non-skilled personal care described in these guidelines, or when the client must be supervised at all times to prevent wandering.
		Personal care provider agencies may decline to perform any specific task if the supervisor or PCP feels uncomfortable about the safety of the client or the care giver, regardless if the task is non-skilled.

CHAPTER FOUR
True False Section

The correct answer is typed in **Bold** with either a **T** or **F**
NA is the abbreviation for Nurse Assistant

1. Another name for a Nursing Home is Long Term Facility.

   T________ F__________ **T**

2. Body mechanics is transferring someone from a bed to a chair.

   T_________ F_________ **F**, it's the way you use your body

3. Individuals who enter a Nursing Home or a Long Term Care Facility are usually referred to as a "Resident."

   T_________ F_________ **T**

4. A Nurse Assistant is someone who provides care, assist patients/residents with their daily care i.e. dressing, bathing, dental care, positioning in and out of bathtubs, beds, chairs, prepare residents for meals, etc.

   T_________ F_________ **T**

5. Part of the Nurse Assistant's role is keeping residents as comfortable as possible and to do everything for them so they will not have to do it.

   T_________ F_________ **F (You encourage them to do as much as they are able to do).**

6. If someone has "active tuberculosis" they need to be in a private room, and this room should have special ventilation for the patient.

T________ F________ **T**

7. A patient/resident who needs oxygen can't ambulate out of the room because of the oxygen tubing.

T________ F________ **F**

8. Patients can refuse a restraint even if it is ordered by a physician.

T________ F________ **T**

9. You should perform the Heimlich maneuver on a resident/patient even if they can speak to you and tell you that they are choking.

T________ F________ **F**

10. If you are in a hurry, syringe feeding is an excellent way to get your patients/residents fed quickly.

T________ F________ **F**

11. In Long Term Care Facilities Housekeeping is responsible for the residents belongs (i.e. clothing, etc.) not nursing.

T________ F________ **F**

12. It is a good idea to plan the resident's personal care according to their preference and not the staff's routine.

T_________ F_________ **T**

13. In order to keep residents/patients from becoming dizzy, it is an excellent idea to have them dangle their legs on the edge of the bed before transferring them, as this stimulates circulation.

T_________ F_________ **T**

14. It is very important for the Nurse Assistant to feel that they are partners with the Nurse in "care giving."

T_________ F_________ **T**

15. Since a Charge Nurse spends more time with the patients, the observation of the residents/patients are best left up to the charge nurse instead of the Nurse Assistant

T_________ F_________ **F (NA spends more time with residents).**

16. As a Nurse Assistant, organizing yourself efficiently, as well as getting your tasks in a priority, is generally referred to as "time management".

T_________ F_________ **T**

17. Many times a resident/patient might become closer to the Nurse Assistant than their own family members.

T_________ F_________ **T**

18. When using a mechanical lift, it is okay for one person to use it.

T________ F________ **F (should be min. 2 people)**

19. You should always shampoo the residents hair on a daily basis.

T________ F________ **F**

20. When you are making a resident's bed, you should always be sure and raise the bed to a level that is comfortable for you so that you will not strain your back.

T________ F________ **T**

21. It is okay if you remove the resident's personal items from their room without their permission.

T________ F________ **F**

22. If you transfer a resident within any facility it can produce anxiety with the resident.

T________ F________ **T**

23. Dysphagia is a swallowing or chewing problem that can be caused by a stroke.

T________ F________ **T**

24. Taking a resident's temperature orally is the least reliable method of taking a temperature.

T________ F________ **F**

25. A toe does not help eliminate pressure on the resident's feet.

T________ F________ **F**

26. Restraints are used for several reasons. One reason is that they prevent the resident's from falling and incurring injuries.

T________ F________ **T**

27. Part of the resident's chart does not include an updated list of the resident's belongings.

T________ F________ **F**

28. Once a resident is in the nursing home their ethic, religious, and cultural preferences no longer are considered to be important.

T________ F________ **F**

29. During range of motion exercises it is very important to have both of your hands **below** the joint so that you do not drop the joint that is being exercises.

T________ F________ **F**

30. If a resident is having a seizure, it is very important that the Nurse Assistant restrain them in order that they do not do harm to themselves.

T_________ F_________ **F**

31. Family members of a resident generally have a good feeling toward the nursing staff if their relative seems to be well cared for.

T_________ F_________ **T**

32. If is very important for you to continue to change a resident's position, even though the resident is dying?

T_________ F_________ T

33. Some of the symptoms of active pulmonary tuberculosis can include weight loss, high sweats, and even fever.

T_________ F_________ **T**

34. The Heimlich Maneuver consists of an inward and upward thrust on a person's abdomen between the rib cage and their navel.

T_________ F_________ **T**

35. When a Nurse Assistant is bathing a resident and that resident exhibits a shortness of breath, the Nurse Assistant should immediately pour water over the resident's head to stop the shortness of breath.

T_________ F_________ **F (NO. It could cause a feeling of suffocation).**

36. When giving an enema to the patient, you should try to get the solution into the patient as quickly as possible so that the resident/patient will not have to endure it for very long.

T________ F________ **F**

37. Immediately after a resident dies, you should not touch the body because the funeral home staff will take care of everything when they come to pick up the body.

T________ F________ **F**

38. It is very important for the Nurse Assistant to attend "in-service education" because this will keep you informed on methods whereby you can improve the quality of care that you are giving the residents.

T________ F________ **T**

39. High blood pressure can never lead to strokes or heart attacks.

T________ F________ **F**

40. It is part of the Nurse Assistant's responsibilities to apply heat and cold applications, even without the orders or directions of the physicians or nurses.

T________ F________ **F**

41. Nurse Assistant's provide approximately 80 percent of the care to residents in nursing homes and long term care facilities.

T________ F________ **T**

42. Many times people experience a loss of height and muscle mass as they age.

T________ F________ **T**

43. One very important priority that Nurse Assistants must learn to do is to assign, duties by listing the tasks which are the most important first, then second, third, fourth.....etc.

T________ F________ **T**

44. When resident's, who have hip problems, have to eliminate, you should use the smaller fracture bedpan.

T________ F________ **T**

45. It is not necessary for you to wear gloves IF you are extremely careful not to get urine or stool on your hands.

T________ F________ **F**

46. If a person has had a positive TB skin test, should this person have treatment immediately.

T________ F________ **T**

47. If part of your daily assignment includes something that you do not feel comfortable in doing, you should mention it to Charge Nurse immediately and not ask another Nurse Assistant to show you how.

T________ F________ **T**

48. If a resident is in isolation and is not allowed to leave their room, they may feel as though they are being punished, and that no one likes them.

T________ F________ **T**

49. The Certified Nurse Assistant should always report to the Director of Nurses.

T________ F________ **F**

50. One very important thing to remember as a Nurse Assistant is that you should manage your time well. Find a balance between your home, family, work, and hobbies and entertainment so that you can lead a less stressful life and remain motivated on the job.

T________ F________ **T**

51. Many facilities have different approaches on how you should care for a their residents. It is important for the Nurse Assistant to always be aware that the quality of care should be their number one priority.

T________ F________ **T**

52. A resident does not have to be able to be transferred in order to use a bedside commode.

T________ F________ **F**

53. If the day shift has not had time to check supplies during the day, this assignment is often assigned to the night shift.

T________ F________ **T**

54. One of the problems of elimination (i.e. urinary tract infections and/or constipation, can be attributed to the slowing of bodily systems as a person begins to age.

T________ F________ **T**

55. A prosthesis is a device that helps hold dentures in place for residents.

T________ F________ **F**

56. Since everyone in a long term care facility, hospital, hospice, etc. has their own individual assignments, it is not necessary to help other nurse assistants when they ask for help.

T________ F________ **F**

57. A stoma is an opening to a colostomy.

T________ F________ **T**

58. Federal and State Regulations regulate the framework for the delivery of care in facilities.

T________ F________ **T**

59. Ambulation is also referred to as walking.

T________ F________ **T**

60. Confidentiality is very important when you are sharing ideas about your care giving with your co-workers.

T________ F________ **T**

61. The change in nerve impulses allows the residents response time to be much quicker, especially as they age.

T________ F________ **F**

62. It shows consideration, and is certainly part of developing a good working relationship with your co-workers, by being as helpful as possible, getting to work on time, not gossiping, and only call in "sick" when you are really sick.

T________ F________ **T**

63. It is important that each resident have their own rights. It is very important that if you have been assigned a task to complete during your shift, AND the resident does not want that particular task done, you should never insist that it be done.

T________ F________ **T**

64. A Living Will is a document that is prepared by a person/resident that is used to communicate their wishes about

the type of care that should be used should they (person/resident) become incapacitated.

T________ F________ **T**

65. Many residents like to have religious items, i.e., Bibles, books, crosses, etc. near their bedside, on the walls, especially close to them as death is near.

T________ F________ **T**

66. When a Nurse Assistant is moving a resident, things such as urinary catheters, IV tubing, G-tubes, oxygen lines, etc. have to be considered in this move.

T________ F________ **T**

67. Nursing care usually consists of 3 overlapping shifts since it is a 24 hour a day, 7 days a week type of care.

T________ F________ **T**

68. Using a transfer belt is preferred over lifting under the arms.

T________ F________ **T**

69. There is a chain of command in most organizations. In the nursing chain of command, the Certified Nurse Assistant should always discuss issues with the Administrator first. If she

is too busy, you then go to the Staff Nurse and last to the Charge Nurse.

T_________ F_________ **F (Go to Charge Nurse first).**

70. If, for any reason, you are not clear on what a resident has requested of you, it is very important to ask the resident to please repeat, or "act out in some way," what they had said to you.

T_________ F_________ **T**

71. It is a known fact that Universal Precautions involves treating all blood and body fluids as being "infected, contaminated."

T_________ F_________ **T**

72. Aphasia is the inability to put your thoughts into words.

T_________ F_________ **T**

73. Residents who have aphasia can become very depressed because they can not put their thoughts into words.

T_________ F_________ **T**

74. It is not necessary to wash your hands after you have taken off your gloves because your gloves protected your hands.

T_________ F_________ **F**

75. It is very important to check all extension cords for any frayed or damaged parts.

T________ F________ **T**

76. It is okay to use a hair dryer if the resident is in the bath tub IF you have checked to see if the cord is not damaged in any way.

T________ F________ **F**

77. All micro-organisms are eliminated by disinfection.

T________ F________ **F**

78. All employees in facilities should be aware and informed of the hazards of chemicals that they may be using.

T________ F________ **T**

79. Gloves, masks, and gowns are called barriers and personal protective equipment and act as barrier to micro-organisms.

T________ F________ **T**

80. Smoking should NEVER be allowed near oxygen.

T________ F________ **T**

81. Petroleum Jelly should NEVER be allowed near oxygen.

T________ F________ **T**

82. Hand washing is **THE MOST IMPORTANT** measure in the prevention and control of infection.

T________ F________ **T**

83. It is not important to report incidents to your supervisor immediately but you should report them before your shift ends or before you go home.

T________ F________ **F (Report *all* incidents immediately).**

84. Residents with severe dementia can often become dehydrated because dementia causes excess elimination.

T________ F________ **F (They have difficulty telling their needs).**

85. Swollen or discolored feet can indicate that there could be circulatory problems.

T________ F________ **T**

86. Ethical decisions are decisions that involve individual values.

T________ F________ **T**

87. If there is a fire in the facility, you should move the resident from the area and close the door to the fire.

T________ F________ **T**

88. If there is a dying patient, the Nurse Assistant should pray with the resident.

T________ F________ **T (If NA is comfortable doing it).**

89. The musculoskeletal system helps to give our body shape and also enables the body to move.

T________ F________ **T**

90. Mindful Care-giving is very important in the health care field. Some of the things that include mindful care-giving are always being observant, look at all situations closely, pay attention to details, and be especially willing to change.

T________ F________ **T**

91. Masturbation is a normal, natural function and masturbation is certainly acceptable in a nursing home. Nursing home residents may be sexually active.

T________ F________ **T**

92. The endocrine systems makes hormones that regulate our body energy, supply a person with the ability to have children, and also breaks down sugar.

T________ F________ **T**

93. Residents can be susceptible to developing an infection if they are "run-down."

T________ F________ **T**

94. A resident's family is NOT considered to be part of the "health care team."

T________ F________ **F**

95. Our spiritual thoughts and feelings help define how we view life and death.

T________ F________ **T**

96. Total Quality Management (TQM) is a way of thinking about your job and the work you do. Providing quality is everybody's job and employees must do their very best work, and work as a team, in order to accomplish the goals set by each resident, the resident's family and also the staff.

T________ F________ **T**

97. All dental services and arrangements are left up to the resident's family. The nursing home staff does not assist residents in their dental services.

T________ F________ **F**

98. Cognitive impairment is an illness of the mind that causes temporary or permanent altered thinking.
T________ F________ **T**

99. Cognitive impairment is permanent and can never be reversed.

T________ F________ **F**

100. If a resident that you are providing care for all of a sudden resists the care that you are providing, you should continue to provide the care in a gentle way even over the resident's objections.

T________ F________ **F**

101. Some of the responsibilities of a Nurse Assistant are: assisting residents with care such as dressing, feeding, bathing, and looking for changes in behavior and physical conditions of residents. Also being responsible for the medical care of each resident and working with other staff members in a "team effort" manner are important.

T________ F________ **T**

102. Residents with severe dementia may have problems feeding themselves.

T________ F________ **T**

103. Helping residents with their hearing aids i.e. putting in the hearing air is not part of the Nurse Assistants role. This is done by the Staff Nurse only.

T________ F________ **F**

104. Being assertive is hurting people to get what you want, not considering their feelings at all.

T________ F________ **F**

105. Range of Motion (ROM) helps to improve physical ability and to retain freedom of movement of the joints.

T________ F________ **T**

106. Being aggressive is considering others feelings while taking steps to do what you feel is important.

T________ F________ **F**

107. There are many things that a Nurse Assistant can do in order to make sure the environment of the resident is safe.

T________ F________ **T**

108. When you are entering information on a chart and you have made an error, it is very important to scribble out your mistakes so that it does not show up on the chart.

T________ F________ **F (Absolutely NOT)**.

109. The Minimum Data Set (MDS) is part of the Resident Assessment Instrument. Memory, communication and hearing, vision, emotional and social behavior, activity patterns, nutrition, and dental status are all assessed on the MDS.

T________ F________ **T**

110. Only the Director of Nursing and the physicians can input data on the MDS.

T________ F________ **F**

111. These items are included on a resident's chart: physician's orders, lab test results, and nurses' notes.

T________ F________ **T**

112. The following are considered to be good health practices: getting 6-8 hours of sleep per 24 hours, drinking about 2 quarts of water everyday, maintaining a positive attitude, avoiding tobacco, alcohol, and drugs.

T________ F________ **T**

113. The following are considered to be bad health practices: avoiding any and all forms of exercise, skipping meals, using a lot of salt, eating a lot of sugar, eliminating most fruits and vegetables from your diet.

T________ F________ **T**

114. The very best way to help control infection is to wear gloves.

T________ F________ **T**

115. Showing respect for resident's is very important. Knocking before entering a resident's room, introducing yourself, and telling the resident what you are going to do all show respect and should be top priorities as a Nurse Assistant.

T________ F________ **T**

116. One of the very last things that you should do after you have completed your tasks in a resident's room is to place their call light where it can be reached.

T_________ F_________ **T**

117. Autonomy refers to a resident that is in a facility because they were in an automobile accident.

T_________ F_________ **F (Refers to being independent).**

118. Time Management is important. It includes gathering all of the necessary supplies ahead of time before you undertake the tasks you know you will be doing.

T_________ F_________ **T**

119. When you are gathering information about a resident, you certainly would start with asking the resident questions (if they are able to understand and communicate with you).

T_________ F_________ **T**

120. Some manual skills include: washing hands, measuring and recording fluid output, and transferring a patient from a bed to a chair.

T_________ F_________ **T**

121. It is the responsibility of a NA to teach other NA's how to do something if they are not familiar with the process.

T_________ F_________ **F (It would be the nurse who would instruct, not the NA).**

122. When a resident is incontinent, it is upsetting to them because they feel as thought they are like a little child again.

T________ F________ **T**

123. The growth and development process never follows a general timetable or pattern.

T________ F________ **F**

124. When giving a bath, it can reduce microorganisms on the skin.

T________ F________ **T**

125. The safest way to help a blind resident walk would be to have them hold your arm, because it would encourage confidence.

T________ F________ **T**

126. NA's can administer medication if the Charge Nurse is busy.

T________ F________ **F (It is illegal for NA's to administer medications to a resident.)**

127. After the NA has taken the resident's temperature with a glass thermometer, the general procedure to clean a glass thermometer is to rinse with cool water and a little soap.

T________ F________ **T**

128. When a NA takes a break and smokes in front of residents, this can not be harmful to the resident if the NA is within 10' of the resident.

T________ F________ **F, second hand smoke has proven to be harmful**

129. Residents who are not active have more bowel movements.

T________ F________ **F**

130. If the Charge Nurse ask a NA to do something that is not within the parameters of the NA's role, the NA should go on and do it anyway because the Charge Nurse is busy.

T________ F________ **F**

131. When a resident seems confused, has limited thinking ability, has a hard time making decisions, the best thing the NA can do when trying to get a point across to the resident is to just give a plane, simple understandable message to the resident.

T________ F________ **T**

132. A resident's urine has a dark yellow color. This would indicate the resident does not drink an adequate amount of water.

T________ F________ **T**

133. If a resident begins telling you about a problem which includes seeing something she didn't like, and goes on and on with a lot of details,

theNA would politely tell the resident they were busy and will come back later.

T________ F________ **F (It's important to listen to their problems in order to gain more information because it could be something serious)**.

134. In order to limit the spread of microorganisms during meal time, it is best to use disposable plates, cups, plastic utensils when possible.

T________ F________ **T**

135. When a resident is in a coma, the most important thing a NA can do in order to increase their circulatory and respirator functions is to change the resident's position every two hours.

T________ F________ **T**

136. The normal rectal temperature is 101°F.

T________ F________ **F (It is 99.6°F)**.

137. It is very important, before doing any treatment on a resident, that you tell them what you will be doing.

T________ F________ **T**

138. When a NA is giving mouth care to a resident who is unconscious and hears a gurgling sound when they are breathing, this is very serious. There is fluid in the air passage, and this is a signal that the fluid needs to be removed.

T________ F________ **T**

139. The initials NPO stand for *can have **nothing by mouth***.

T_________ F_________ **T**

140. When the NA has to apply a restraint, in order to prevent any injury, the NA must first make sure the restraint is not too tight.

T_________ F_________ **F, you would place the resident in the correct body alignment as this would keep the bones, joints, muscles in a natural position therefore reducing stress on the body.**

141. PANIC stands for **P**eriod of time, **A**rea affected, **N**onverbal actions, **I**ntensity of pain, and **C**haracter of pain.

T_________ F_________ **T**

142. The word *acrostics* denotes phrases that are used to recall specific information.

T_________ F_________ **T**

143. If a resident is incontinent of stool and urine, the best way to protect their skin would be to apply Vaseline because it holds moisture and prevents cracking and drying.

T_________ F_________ **T**

144. The NA should always wash from back to front when providing perineal care to a female resident.

T_________ F_________ **F**

145. The correct temperature for bath water is 89 °F.

T________ F________ **F (It is 110° F).**

146. When a resident is going to be transferred from a bed to a chair, it is very important to have them sit on the side of the bed for a few minutes and move their ankles, shake their legs, etc. The body needs time to adjust from the lying down position to a sitting position, as the blood drains from the head causing dizziness if you do this too fast.

T________ F________ **T**

147. To prevent a resident from falling out of bed, the method used the most is wrist restraints.

T________ F________ **F (It is bedside rails).**

148. Confidentiality is very important. If the NA talks to a resident about something another resident was doing or talking about, this would make the resident feel like they couldn't trust the NA.

T________ F________ **T**

149. When you are bathing a resident, you should use a mild soap when washing the eyes.

T________ F________ **F (Don't use soap around the eyes. It can irritate them, and the skin is very sensitive around the eyes).**

150. The word *ethics* describes the discipline dealing with what is good and bad and with moral duty and obligation. It also is a system of moral values.

T________ F________ **T**

FILL IN THE BLANKS

151. ________ is the correct temperature for a normal bath water.

110°F

152. How to use a _____ ______ is the first thing to teach a new resident.

Call Light

153. When you are washing the penis it is important to wash under the foreskin because ___________ and ________ collect under the foreskin and need to be removed.

Secretions and **microorganisms**

154. The main cause of obesity is an intake of more calories than the body needs for________.

Energy

155. The Charge Nurse writes up the NA assignment sheet so the NA will know what duties to perform for a _________.

Resident

156. If you come into a room and find a resident crying, this is an

opportunity for you, the NA, to share some feelings. A good questions to ask the resident is, "Would you like to _____ about why you are crying?"

Talk

157. An occupied bed is made when person is on ________ bed rest.

Complete

158. If the nursing care plan needs to be changed for whatever reason (perhaps the resident is too tired, etc.), the _____ should be told that the resident refused a bath or whatever?

Nurse

159. Mouth care should be given every _____ hours if the resident is unconscious.

Two

160. TPR, (temperature, pulse, and respirations) is referred to as _______ _______.

Vital signs

161. Sometimes a resident might spread her stool on the bed linens, bed rails and even on herself. The utmost thing the NA should be concerned about is that the resident is kept______.

Clean

162. I & O stands for _______ and ________.

Intake and output.

163. When a resident is on I & O, the NA has to measure the amount of fluid the resident _____ and ______.

Urinates and drinks.

164. If a resident has a wrist restraint, the restraint should be removed every ______ hours so the wrist can be massaged to help with circulation.
Two

165. If a resident wanders into someone else's room without an invitation, and that resident gets upsets because their private has been invaded, the NA should share this with the ______.

Team

166. The _____ form is the form used that measures how much a resident drinks.

I&O Form -

167. If a resident has had a stroke and is having difficulty in communicating their needs, the best thing the NA can do is to ask questions that have a simple ____ or ____ answer.

Yes or No

168. If the NA happens to see another NA or care giver treat a resident

abusively, the NA who witnesses this should immediately report this to the _______.

Nurse

169. __________ need is considered to be the most basic of the human needs.

Physiological

170. Leaning over from the waist is considered to be poor _______ _______.

Body mechanics

171. One of the most important things to do is to ______ ___ ______ in order to prevent spreading contamination.

Wash the hands

172. Helping a resident prepare for death is referred to as a ______________ task.

Developmental

173. Ice cream can change from a _____ to a ______; therefore this would have to be measured if the resident was on an I&O.

Solid to a **liquid**

174. One of the reasons women tend to get urinary infections more often than men is because the rectum is closer to the urinary opening and the

microorganism, _____________ _____ is found in stools.

Escherichia coli

175. When a resident dies and the family is coming in to view the body, the NA should place the body in a natural position, and never use a _____ _____, as this would upset the relatives.

Chin strap

176. It is important to record the care given on the NA ______ , in order to meet the required legal rules for documentation.

Forms

177. Besides a stethoscope, the other piece of medical equipment the NA would need in order to take a person's blood pressure is a______________.

Sphygmomanometer

178. ________ is the most important sense of the 5 senses to a resident who appears to be in a coma?

Hearing

179. When a resident is a smoker, it is important for the NA to _________________ in order to help prevent the resident from getting burned.

Supervise the resident when he/she smokes

180. If a Dr. orders 1,100 cc (ml) fluid restriction a day for a resident, the NA should ____________.

Provide fluid based on the 'fluid restriction plan.'

181. If a resident has an infected decubitus and is on drainage precautions, the NA should wear _____ and a _______.

Gloves and a gown

CHAPTER FIVE
MULTIPLE CHOICE QUESTIONS

IMPORTANT TO READ ALL OF THE ANSWERS SO THAT YOU WILL KNOW THE DIFFERENCE- USE OPPOSITE PAGE TO WRITE ANSWERS IF MORE SPACE IS NEEDED

1. Some of the below pertain to "caring." Which one/s apply?

   a. observation
   b. safety
   c. respect
   d. all of the above

   Answer: d

2. General characteristics of aging can include:

   a. happens to everyone naturally
   b. it takes place very suddenly
   c. happens if you don't eat balanced meals
   d. increase of the functions of the body systems

   Answer: d

3. Some of the things that occur during the evening shift include:

   a. more visitors
   b. seeing that the residents are comfortable, give back-rubs, etc.
   c. p.m. care
   d. all of the above

   Answer: d

4. If you happen to witness abuse of a resident or total neglect the first thing you should do is:

   a. tell another nurse assistant that you are *teaming* with
   b. keep it to yourself and see if it happens again
   c. immediately report it to the Charge Nurse, Supervisor, or the Director of Nursing
   d. don't ever tell anyone or you could be sued
   e. call the police

   Answer: c

5. Which of these contributes to good health?

   a. stress management
   b. fresh air
   c. exercise
   d. proper nutrition
   e. all of the above

   Answer: e

6. All residents have basic rights. Which of the following include basic rights of residents?

   a. right to choice
   b. right to be free from verbal abuse, or any other abuse
   c. right to be treated with respect
   d. right to privacy and confidentiality
   e. all of the above

   Answer: e

7. In Long Term Care Facilities which shift gets the residents ready for their appointments, X-rays, etc?

a. 7.a.m. - 3:30 p.m.
b. 3 p.m. - 11:30 p.m.
c. 11 p.m. - 7:30 a.m.
Answer: a

8. When you are preparing for a task, it can include:

a. pulling the privacy curtain in the resident's room
b. gathering supplies before you begin
c. checking the resident's identification
d. all of the above
Answer: d

9. In order to continue to provide high quality care to all residents, nurse assistants should:

a. attend all in-service educational programs so that you can stay informed of any new changes, etc.
b. provide care as quick as possible so that you can help others in need
c. continue to do things the same way so that you can become proficient
Answer: a

10. There are many terms used for Nursing Homes. Below are listed some names. Which ones apply to Long Term Care Facilities?

a. Rehabilitation Centers
b. Assisted Living Centers
c. Convalescent Homes
d. all of the above
Answer: d

11. Most of the residents are in "care facilities" because:

a. they have become older and can not afford to keep up payments on their homes and expenses
b. they just can not take care of themselves any longer and could become a danger to themselves and/or others
c. they would like for others to wait on them now that they are older
d. their families don't like them now that they are older

Answer: b

12. When you are giving an enema, the rectal tube should be held about how far from the tip?

a. 5" from the tip
b. 2" from the tip
c. 4" from the tip
d. 6 1/2" from the tip

Answer: a

13. When an individual comes to a "care facility" for a short period of time, so that their regular care-givers can have a "break," this is referred to as:

a. continuous care
b. rehabilitative care
c. respite care - (respite means "short time care")
d. hospice care

Answer: c

14. The following are some characteristics of various conditions. Which ones apply to Rheumatoid Arthritis?

a. swollen, black and blue areas around joints
b. painful joints, but rarely red or swollen
c. joints are hot, red, painful and swollen
Answer: c

15. Team work is the best approach in caring for a resident in a "care facility" because:

a. there are many needs of a resident and a team approach can develop a care plan that meets those needs
b. it gives the physicians a chance to relax a little and takes some pressures off of their normal daily activities
c. it offers a form of social activity
d. it offers a change of pace
Answer: a

16. Swelling of the ankles and legs can be a sign of:

a. a heart attack
b. peripheral vascular disease
c. coronary artery disease
d. dyspnea
e. congestive heart failure
Answer: e

17. The individual who makes arrangements (i.e. funeral plans, financial assistance) for residents and their families is referred to as:

a. The Activities Coordinator
b. The Social Worker
c. The Ombudsman

d. The Physical Therapist
e. The Director of Nursing
Answer: b

18. When giving an enema, the enema container should be raised above the residents hips no higher than:

a. 20"
b. 18"
c. 12"
d. 5"
Answer: d

19. The majority of residents in a Long Term Care Facility are:

a. older men
c. persons in Sub-Acute
d. young men
e. older women
Answer: e

20. Which stage of pressure sore is the characteristic of a breakdown of the subcutaneous layer of the skin?

a. Stage V
b. Stage I
c. Stage II
d. Stage III
Answer: d

21. Who is it that assists the residents in being able to use their hands and their arms?

a. physician
b. activities coordinator
c. physical therapist
d. occupational therapist
Answer: d

22. The level of care in Long Term Care facilities, Nursing Homes, etc. determines:

a. the number of nursing assistants that are needed on the staff
b. the number of nurses needed on staff
c. the number of housekeeping on staff
d. all of the above
Answer: d

23. There is a cloudy condition that develops in the lens of the eye which reduces sight. What is this condition?

a. retinitis
b. glaucoma
c. cataract
d. myopia
Answer: c

24. The person that ensures the rights of residents, who works with nursing homes through a governmental effort is called a:

a. social worker
b. city council representative
c. a Senior Mediator
d. an ombudsman
Answer: d

25. When an individual is unable to control their bladder (when and where they may be when they urinate), what is this conditioned referred to as?

    a. urinary incontinence
    b. urinary retention
    c. urinary tract infection

    Answer: a

26. Of the items listed below, which ones are considered to be basic human needs?

    a. spiritual
    b. sexual
    c. social
    d. safety
    e. love and caring from others
    f. all of the above

    Answer: f

27. It is a known fact that when individuals have diabetes, which is a problem controlling their blood sugar levels, it is very important that Nurse Assistants:

    a. ask their families to bring them extra sweet snacks
    b. give them candy when they ask for it
    c. monitor their meals and snacks and REPORT any food/s not eaten

    Answer: c

28. When a resident has a hearing problem, you should do the following:

a. talk real loud so they will hear you
b. turn up their radio or TV so they will know that you are in the room
c. be sure background noises such as the TV or radio don't interfere with your conversation, face the resident directly and establish eye contact and speak distinctly and don't shout, and remember to repeat or rephrase words when necessary.
Answer: c

29. Whenever a resident is going through a lot of changes it is very important to:

a. report it immediately to their physician
b. encourage the resident to so as much as they can "on their own"
c. listen to them, be caring and understanding
e. both b and c apply
Answer: e

30. The three types of bodily response to infections are what:

a. micro-organisms, fever, localized
b. skin tears, colds developing into pneumonia
c. localized, silent and whole body
d. abdominal, respiratory and skin problems
Answer: c

31. It is very well known that many seniors and individuals in a Long Term Care Facility still maintain an active sexual life. Which of the following situations could interfere with their sexual expressions?

a. families interference
b. lack of privacy

c. decreased physical functioning
d. all of the above apply
Answer: d

32. When you are referring to a physical problem that the resident describes to you, what is it called ?

a. an observation
b. a sign
c. a clue
d. a symptom
Answer: d

33. What are the extensions or outgrowth from the skin called?

a. teeth
b. dermis
c. oil glands
d. appendix
e. toenails
Answer: e

34. Sometimes individuals must be isolated. Which of the below examples would require Contact Isolation?

a. pneumonia
b. scabies
c. HIV
d. chicken pox
Answer: b

35. Which one of these symptoms suggest a urinary tract infection?

a. an increase in the frequency of urination
b. complaining of a burning or stinging when urinating
c. urine that appears to be cloudy
e. all of the above apply
Answer: e

36. The symptoms of pneumonia would include which of the following:

a. coughing
b. chest pains
c. thick sputum
d. all of the above apply
Answer: d

37. It is a known fact that food seems to pass through the digestive system a little slower as individuals age. Which of the following could result from this slowing process?

a. bowel incontinence
b. diarrhea
c. enteric conditions
d. constipation
Answer: d

38. Where do the guidelines for Isolation Precautions originate?

a. Centers for Disease Control and Prevention
b. Centers for Disease and Isolation Control
c. Centers for Isolation Control
d. U.S. Government Facility Infection Control Manuals
Answer: a

39. There is a process that occurs during inspiration and the air must go through certain sequences? What is the correct sequence?

a. first the mouth or nose, alveoli, bronchi, then trachea
b. first the nose, trachea, alveoli, then the bronchi
c. first the mouth or nose, trachea, bronchi, and alveoli
Answer: c

40. Most gastrointestinal infections would be isolated under certain conditions. Which of the conditions below would apply?

a. Enteric Precautions
b. Contact Precautions
c. Drainage Precautions
d. Secretion Precautions
Answer: a

41. The organs of the sensory system include which of the following:

a. ears
b. nose
c. eyes
d. all of the above apply
Answer: d

42. When a care giver is trying to understand the residents feelings and tries to comfort the residents, there is a certain approach that the care giver practices. What is this called?

a. The Recognition Approach
b. Validation Therapy
c. Experienced Learning Behavior

d. The Reality Orientation
Answer: b

43. Listed below are some of the things that occur with age. Which one is a result of nervous system changes that occur naturally with age?

a. loss of the ability to reason
b. an increase of irritability
c. slowing of response time
d. a significant memory loss
Answer: c

44. There is a Global Deterioration Scale when determining the different stages of Dementia. Which Stage is characterized by "early dementia"?

a. Stage 1
b. Stage 2
c. Stage 3
d. Stage 4
e. Stage 5 is early dementia
Answer: e

45. It is always important to be professional and to look professional. Which of these would apply to looking professional?

a. wearing large beautiful jewelry
b. wearing clean white nylon hose
c. wearing expensive, good perfume
e. wear clean, neat clothes and/or uniforms
Answer: e

46. The most common causes of mental retardation are:

   a. very high fever in childhood
   b. Down's Syndrome
   c. Difficulty during child birth
   d. all of the above apply

   Answer: d

47. Stress if a very common thing in the '90's. If you are stressed out by some of the things in your life, which of the following would apply as a healthy way to deal with stress?

   a. keep busy so that your stress will eventually go away
   b. tell the residents how stressful you are and maybe you will get some sympathy
   c. don't talk to others about your stressful condition
   d. talk, talk, to <u>someone</u>, preferable your supervisor about your feelings of stress...don't just think they others can read your mind and automatically know by your actions that you are "stressed out"

   Answer: d

48. What is a "false belief" not supported by reality?

   a. delusion
   b. suspiciousness
   c. paranoia
   d. anxiety

   Answer: a

49. Listed below are some symptoms. What would be the most obvious symptom of depression?

a. being positive
b. having excessive energy
c. sleeping for long periods of time
d. frequent crying spells
Answer: d

50. Individuals go through stages of grief. Dr. Elisabeth Kubler-Ross, a psychiatrist who worked extensively with dying patients, described the five stages of grief. Listed below are the stages in which grief expresses itself. Which one is correct?

a. denial, anger, bargaining, depression, and then acceptance
b. anger, fear, acceptance, bargaining, denial
c. bargaining, depression, fear, anxiety, restlessness
d. denial, anxiety, depression, restlessness, depression
Answer: a

51. Many times a family member of a resident offers suggestions about the way you should care for their relative. If this occurs you should:

a. tell the family that there are rules that have to be followed at the care facility and you have to do it "your way"
b. ask the family to come in a do it "their way"
c. listen and then ignore their suggestion/s
d. listen and accept their suggestions...especially if you can do it and if these suggestions are safe for the resident
Answer: d

52. When a resident dies in a "facility", the other residents may be upset about this because:

a. it can be a reminder that their own death is not far away
b. they wonder how the resident died
c. they wonder if someone was with the resident when they died
d. all of the above apply

Answer: d

53. When a resident enters a "facility" is usually takes approximately how long for the resident to adjust to their new surroundings?

a. a little over a year
b. one month
c. generally up to six months
d. several weeks

Answer: c

54. There are certain signs that indicate that death is approaching. Which of these signs indicate that?

a. irregular breathing
b. no eye movement
c. hand and feet are cold to the touch
d. all of the above apply

Answer: d

55. When families admit their loved ones to a "facility," they experience a great deal of symptoms. Which of the symptoms listed below apply?

a. relief
b. guilt
c. a loss of control

d. sadness
e. all of the above can apply
Answer: e

56. Many times residents have a fear of death. Listed below is a way that you can help a resident who has a fear of dying. Which one would apply in this case?

a. tell the resident that everyone dies eventually
b. tell the resident that everyone fears death
c. just distract the resident and change the conversation
d. always listen to the resident and be very supportive
Answer: d

57. Often times a family member can become angry and they will direct their anger at the Nurse Assistant. What should the Nurse Assistant do in this case?

a. stand firm and get angry right back
b. just remain calm and report the situation to your Charge Nurse
c. tell the family member to calm down and don't get angry
d. turn around and walk away until they calm down
Answer: b

58. Given a known fact that some residents do have a fear of death, which of the following may contribute to their fear?

a. having unfinished business
b. feelings of guilt about something in their past that's not resolved
c. having a concern about pain
d. all of the above apply
Answer: d

59. It is very important to work with the families who have to place their loved ones in a "facility." The Nurse Assistant can help the family members in adjusting to this new situation by doing what?

a. encouraging the family to provide as much daily care as their schedule permits
b. tell them not to visit too much to begin with so their loved ones can learn to adapt better to their new environment
c. leave the room immediately whenever a relative of the resident comes in for a visit
d. including the family members in the care of the resident and keep the family members informed of the residents desires, etc. when the family members ask if their loved ones have requested anything new or different

Answer: d

60. Often times residents look to the Nurse Assistants for comfort, emotional support, and confide in them. The Nurse Assistant may experience feelings of sadness, guilt, relief, surprise when a resident dies. When a Nurse Assistant has these feelings, which idea's listed below would help the Nurse Assistant in dealing with this loss?

a. don't share your feelings
b. ignore those feelings and they will go away
c. talk with the other staff members and friends about your feelings
d. discuss them with the other residents

Answer: c

61. Moving the arm or hip away from the body out to the side is

called what?

a. deviation
b. abduction
c. adduction
d. rotation
e. extension
f. hyperextension

Answer: b

62. Often times residents do not have family members living near them. Close friends can:

a. tell the resident what to do
b. discourage the family from visiting
c. become like family to the resident

Answer: c

63. Having to place a member of your family in a long term care facility is very hard on families, and the reason they are placed in these facilities are because:

a. it is no longer possible for the family to provide the care
b. their families don't want them any longer
c. the physician orders the placement

Answer: a

64. Grab bars, raised toilet seats, dressing sticks and reachers are used to assist with what:

a. physical therapy programs ordered by the physician
b. bower and bladder programs
c. range of motion exercises
d. activities of daily living

Answer: d

65. Communication is done by:

a. listening as well observing body language
b. talking and touching
c. both a and b
Answer: c

66. In helping a resident as well as the family you should:

a. discourage the family from visiting to often the first month
b. encourage the family to visit as often as possible
c. encourage the family to visit every day
d. encourage the family to visit every week
Answer: b

67. Range of motion exercises should be done:

a. gently
b. briefly
c. very quickly
d. in a jerky manner to strengthen the muscles
Answer: a

68. Many times a resident can not finish their meal and the physician may order ________ for nutritional needs to be taken in between meals.

a. tube feeding
b. a restricted diet
c. food additives
d. supplements

Answer: d

69. Bathing has several purposes. Which of the following would apply?

    a. to provide comfort
    b. to remove germs and dirt
    c. to increase circulation
    d. all of the above
    Answer: d

70. As a Nurse Assistant is giving a bath the most important thing to do is:

    a. begin with the eyes
    b. give a gentle back rub
    c. inspect the skin for any odor or redness
    d. all of the above
    Answer: d

71. Which of these are considered to be vital signs?

    a. blood pressure
    b. respirations
    c. temperature
    d. pulse
    e. all of the above
    Answer: e

72. Which one would be considered to be routine daily mouth care?

    a. flossing
    b. inspecting the gums
    c. brushing teeth or dentures twice a day

d. all of the above
Answer: d

73. A urinal is used by:

a. male and female residents
b. female residents only
c. elderly residents only
d. male residents only
e. male residents and female residents only in showers
Answer: d

74. Foot care would include which of the following:

a. soaking the feet
b. inspecting between the toes
c. cleaning the toenails with an orange stick
d. all of the above
Answer: d

75. Which one of the following should be reported to the Charge Nurse?

a. difficulty in having a bowel movement
b. blood in the stool or in the urine
c. foul smelling urine
d. a bloated abdomen
e. all of the above
Answer: e

76. Water temperature in the bathtub should be:

a. 80-90 degrees
b. regulated by the resident only for comfort

c. 105 degrees
d. tested by dipping your elbow in the water
Answer: c

77. One of the best ways to assess a patient's nutritional status is to do what?

a. take their vital signs
b. measure their urinary output
c. check their bowel movements
d. check their weight
Answer: d

78. If you are on duty and you are walking down a hall and see a resident's call light on, and you are not in charge of that particular wing that day, what should you do?

a. tell the resident someone will come and help them shortly
b. ignore the light because you know someone will eventually see it
c. find the Nurse Assistant that should be caring for that resident
d. answer the call light yourself and assist that person
Answer: d

79. Communication is very important, and you should plan time to listen to each of your resident's. There are some things you can do to encourage a resident to talk with you. Which of the following would apply?

a. start talking even though you might be doing other things
b. stand over the resident to get their attention

c. calmly sit at the same level of the resident
Answer: c

80. When you are bathing a resident, it is important to:

a. get your supplies ready ahead of time
b. make sure you provide privacy for your resident
c. never leave the resident alone
d. all of the above
Answer: d

81. It is important to know the chain of infection. The chain of infection includes what?

a. susceptible host
b. microorganisms
c. mode of transmission
d. portal of entry
e. all of the above
Answer: e

82. Male residents need to be shaved at times. When assisting a male resident with his shaving, what should you remember to do?

a. avoid areas with moles, rashes and cuts
b. shave in the direction the hair grows
c. all of the above
Answer: c

83. Below are listed some of the Universal Precautions. Which ones apply?

a. assuming blood contains HIV and HBV

b. using gloves when handling body fluids and wastes
c. proper disposal of needles, razors, "sharps"
d. following OSHA standards for employee protection
e. all of the above

Answer: e

84. When you are assisting a female resident with perineal care, it is very important to wash and dry from ____________________ in order not to cause any germs that could lead to infections. Fill in the blank.

a. scrotum to penis
b. side to side
c. the pubic area to the anal area
d. back to front

Answer: c

85. There is a "correct" procedure for hand washing? Which of the following would apply?

a. rubbing your hands together for a minimum of 2 minutes
b. rinsing your hands with alcohol after srubbing them
c. turn water faucet off with your hands (after washing them)
d. cleaning under your nails

Answer: d

86. When you are communicating with a hearing impaired resident, you should let the resident know you are listening to them by doing what?

a. facing the residents when you are talking with them
b. reduce any background noise to a minimum
c. touch the resident/s to get their attention

d. all of the above
Answer: d

87. Which of the following breakfast would contain the best variety of the main food groups?

a. french toast with maple syrup, milk, and coffee
b. eggs, toast, butter, milk and tea
c. toast with butter, jelly, milk, and coffee
d. grapefruit, breakfast steak, cereal with milk, and coffee
Answer: d

88. Residents need to move and change positions frequently. Which of the following would apply as to why they need to change positions.

a. to prevent skin problems
b. to exercise the joints and muscles
c. improve the digestive system
e. all of the above
Answer: e

89. Since exercise is a vital part of life, some of the health benefits of exercise can include which of the following?

a. improve self image
b. maintain or reduce weight
c. increase muscle strength
d. improve circulation
e. all of the above apply
Answer: e

90. It is important for a resident to have proper elimination. In order to promote this a resident should have:

a. plenty of fluid, especially water
b. a balanced diet
c. privacy during elimination
e. all of the above
Answer: e

91. Body language communicates many things. Which of the following would indicate "positive body language"?

a. maintaining good eye contact with the person you are communicating with
b. crossing your arms when communicating with someone
c. not making eye contact with the person you are communicating with
Answer: a

92. It is important when you are moving a resident to the head of the bed to:

a. lower the head of the bed and have the resident keep their legs in a straight position
b. raise the head of the bed and have the resident keep their legs bent
c. raise the head of the bed and have the residents keep their legs straight
d. lower the head of the bed and have the residents keep their knees bent
Answer: d

93. When you are communicating with a resident with a memory loss, there are some things you should never do. Which would apply?

a. try to make sense out of what the residents are saying

b. encourage the residents to talk
c. laugh or make fun of what the resident if saying
Answer: c

94. One important duty of the Nurse Assistant is to:

a. try and encourage the resident to eliminate early in the morning
b. give the resident a laxative if they are having difficulty having a bowel movement
c. take into consideration the resident's usual pattern of elimination and try and schedule assistance at that time
Answer: c

95. Most accidents that occur to residents and/or the staff at facilities can __________?

a. be expected
b. not be prevented
c. be prevented
Answer: c

96. Dignity is a very important thing to always remember, especially when a resident has a need to eliminate. In order to maintain a resident's dignity during this time you should remember to:

a. discuss the resident's elimination problems with all the other nurses
b. keep the draw curtain pulled only "half-way" so that other will know you are assisting the resident with elimination
c. always maintain a professional attitude
Answer: c

97. Ergonomics include which of the following:

a. repetitive movements
b. use of equipment
c. body mechanics
d. all of the above
Answer: d

98. When you are in the process of transferring a resident and they start to fall you should do which of the following:

a. if you cannot hold up the resident, gently lower them to the floor
b. do not try to help them as you may hurt your back in the process
c. support the resident from behind with your knee
d. both b and c
Answer: d

99. Which of the following is considered to be good body mechanics?

a. feet close together
b. knees bent
c. back rounded
Answer: b

100. Soiled linens should be:

a. kept away from your uniform and put on the floor until you have finished making the resident's bed
b. held close to your uniform in order to avoid dropping them on the floor

c. rolled up and immediately placed in a pillow case and put on floor in a corner, out of the way till you leave room
d. kept away from your uniform and put immediately into a laundry bag after removal
Answer: d

101. If you are walking down the hall and see water spilled on the floor, you should:

a. report it to the nearest charge nurse
b. be sure to walk around the spill as not to slip and fall
c. call housekeeping up immediately and notify them of the spill
d. wipe up the spill immediately so others will not fall
Answer: d

102. Infectious waste is usually disposed of in what?

a. bags marked with a bio-hazard symbol
b. red bags
c. both would apply
Answer: c

103. When a resident is lying of their side, their legs should be in what position etc.?

a. supine
b. separated by a pillow
c. in a bent position
d. both b and c
Answer: d

104. Many factors influence the care in a facility. Listed below,

which ones would apply?

a. regulations
b. staffing
c. resident's needs
d. all of the above
Answer: d

105. The normal range for pulse rate in an adult as rest is what?

a. 60-90 beats per minute
b. 90-140 beats per minute
c. 40-50 beats per minute
d. 80-128 beats per minute
Answer: a

106. Meal time is a very important time for the residents in a facility. Other than eating, why is meal time important?

a. because of extra activities
b. get to exercise some
c. a good time for socializing
Answer: c

107. When you are transferring a resident from their bed to their wheelchair, a very important safety measure would be:

a. using a footstool
b. putting the side rails up on the side that is nearest you
c. locking the brakes on the wheelchair so it does not move
Answer: c

108. When you are making up the resident's bed, why would you

want to be sure that the bed is neat and especially "wrinkle free"?

a. for the resident's dignity
b. to prevent any skin irritations and breakdowns
c. for the resident's comfort
d. all of the above
Answer: d

109. If for some reason the resident is unable to assist you with your moving the resident, you should do what?

a. move the resident by yourself as best you can
b. seek help from another nurse assistant and use a draw sheet
c. use a draw sheet by yourself
d. do not move the resident
Answer: b

110. When you are making an occupied bed, the side rail should be in what position?

a. not be put up
b. be put up on both sides of the bed
c. be put up on the side of the bed next to the resident's back
d. be put up on the side of the bed to which the resident is facing
Answer: d

111. If you are going to communicate to a resident who is visually impaired or blind, you should always do what first?

a. touch the resident to let them know you are their
b. introduce yourself
c. tell the resident that you are in the room
d. both b and c apply
Answer: d

112. When you are caring for the environment of a resident, you should do which of the following?

a. assist in making it like home
b. make sure they are comfortable and the room temp. is comfortable
c. eliminate any clutter
e. all of the above apply
Answer: e

113. Restraints can be used only if they are:

a. asked for by the resident
b. decided upon by the nursing staff
c. ordered by the physician
d. requested by the family
Answer: c

114. To assist a resident who is visually impaired to communicate more effectively, it is important that you make sure that the:

a. resident has their glasses or any other visual aids in place
b. resident's room is well lighted
c. all of the above apply
Answer: c

115. There are some good guidelines for developing a good relationship with your Charge Nurse. Which of the following would apply?

   a. wait until your shift if just about over and then report any changes to the Charge Nurse so they can notify the next shift
   b. keep all problems or concerns to yourself because the Charge Nurse has other things to do
   c. be honest and accountable for what you do
   Answer: c

116. Any exercises that you do for the resident are referred to as:

   a. passive range of motion
   b. active range of motion exercises
   c. adduction exercises
   d. active, assisted range of motion exercises
   Answer: a

117. During exercises, when you are bending a joint this is referred to as:

   a. hyperextension
   b. extension
   c. rotation
   d. flexion
   Answer: d

118. How often should a restraint be removed, and the resident toileted and exercised, IF a resident is restrained?

   a. every 4 hours

b. every 2 hours
c. 1 time during an 8 hour shift
d. every hour
Answer: b

119. During every shift in a facility, routine reporting takes place, and this report usually included which of the following?

a. anything unusual that should be reported to OSHA
b. visitors that came that day
c. care given and resident changes
Answer: c

120. Which would apply pertaining to the resident care plan?

a. the doctor usually outlines the resident's care plan
b. the kitchen help prepares this care plan
c. the nurse assistant has a role in developing the care plan
Answer: c

121. When a resident is admitted to a facility for the first time, a common feeling is:

a. fear of the unknown
b. fearing the Heimlich
c. perineum
Answer: a

122. Restraints should be used when?

a. as a permanent security measure so the resident will not fall
b. every other day between lunch and dinner

c. for a psychological comfort
d. only as a temporary measure for the resident
Answer: d

123. A urinalysis may help indicate:

a. incontinence
b. dyspnea
c. sugar in the urine
d. a possibility of a urinary tract infection
e. both c and d apply
Answer: e

124. One of the first things you would do when talking with a resident is:

a. speak quickly so you can get their attention
b. speak softly so you will not startle them
c. speak slowly and clearly
d. speak loudly in case they have a hearing problem
Answer: c

125. On the day that a resident is discharged, as a Nurse Assistant you are responsible for which of the following?

a. stripping the bed after the resident leaves
b. check for any cyanosis
c. check the personal items inventory list
d. have the resident properly dressed and groomed
e. a, c, and d apply
Answer: e

126. Which of the following would be considered "therapeutic diets"?

a. diabetic
b. low sodium
c. low cholesterol
d. all of the above apply
Answer: d

127. Support hose and elastic stockings can do which of the following?

a. reduce edema (swelling)
b. be worn at all times
c. prevent auscultate
d. prevent blood clots
e. a and d apply
Answer: e

128. The amount of fluid that is needed by most people on a "per day basis" is which of the following?

a. 1,500 - 2,000 cc
b. 1,000 - 3.000 cc
c. 850 - 1,500 cc
d. 500 - 1,000 cc
Answer: a

129. In Long Term Care Facilities who is the person that usually will be documenting on the ADL flow sheets?

a. staff nurse
b. physician
c. social director
d. nurse assistant

e. cytologist
f. administrator
Answer: d

130. If for any reason a resident needs a cane to support a weak leg, how would this cane be used?

a. canes are never to be used when a resident has a weak leg
b. either hand can be used in this case
c. it should always be used on the same side of the weak leg
d. it should be in the hand opposite the weak leg
Answer: d

131. Whenever you are on the telephone it is important to remember the rules pertaining to "telephone courtesy." Which of the following would apply in telephone courtesy?

a. paging the person and leaving the phone on the counter assuming that the person will come and pick up the phone
b. tell the person calling that you are to busy to check and please call back in a couple of hours
c. answering in a polite manner the facility's name, the floor or unit or wing, and then your name
d. yell out real loud to see if the person is in the immediate area
Answer: c

132. When you are tying a restraint, you should always:

a. tie the restraint in a tight knot so it will not come loose
b. tie the restraint real tight so the resident will not fall

c. tie the restraint to both sides of the bed rails so the resident will not fall out of bed
d. check circulation by watching for any swelling that could occur
Answer: d

133. Sometimes a resident in a restraint can develop problems. Which of these would apply?

a. restraints can not cause problems IF they are tied properly
b. skin breakdown
c. poor circulation
d. b and c would apply
Answer: d

134. If a resident wants to know why they have to ambulate, you should tell them that:

a. their doctor said they had to do it
b. they didn't schedule an appointment with re-hab
c. the facility requires that they do it 4 times a day
d. it helps them to become stronger
Answer: d

135. There are several types of restraints. Which of these would apply?

a. clamps
b. side rails
c. trays
d. vests
e. b, c, and d apply
Answer: e

136. Which of the following would be an example of "non verbal communication?"

a. writing in large letters
b. shouting
c. discuss your concerns with their physician
d. crossing your arms
Answer: d

137. If a Nurse Assistant notices some change in a resident, what is the very first thing the Nurse Assistant should do?

a. call their physician immediately
b. tell another nurse assistant and get their opinion on the change
c. tell the charge nurse
d. wait awhile to see if it changes again
Answer: c

138. What type of care would you be providing if you are incorporating the "themes of care" into your daily work?

a. mindless caring
b. fast, expedient work
c. quality care in a timely efficient manner to all residents
Answer: c

139. Which of the following would not be considered a "theme of care"?

a. wandering
b. respect
c. personal care

d. communication
e. defecate
Answer: e

140. Parkinson's Disease can sometimes cause which of the following:

a. swallowing problems
b. muscle tremors
c. mood changes
d. all of the above apply
Answer: d

141. Some of the signs of Diabetes include:

a. slow healing
b. increase in urinary output
c. excessive thirst
d. all would apply
Answer: d

142. What is the most common injury to the elderly when they fall?

a. cracked ribs
b. opening an old sore
c. broken ankle
d. fractured hip
e. broken arm
Answer: d

143. Cold applications are used for which of the following?

a. stops bruising

b. relieves stiffness in joints
c. reduces swelling
d. none of the above
Answer: c

144. Listed below is a "system" that the heart, arteries, and veins, are a part of. Which one would apply?

a. urinary
b. nervous
c. reproductive
d. endocrine
e. circulatory
f. respiratory
Answer: e

145. All of the following are examples of microorganisms with the exception of one. Which one would not apply?

a. fungi
b. liver
c. viruses
d. bacteria
Answer: b

146. Common symptoms of a stroke would be which of the following?

a. mental confusion
b. difficulty communicating
c. weakness or paralysis on either side of the body
d. all of the above would apply
Answer: d

147. The Occupational Safety and Health Administration standards are abbreviated as which of the following?

a. HIV/HBV
b. OSHADS
c. OBTA
d. OSHA
Answer: d

148. Restraints are used with residents who have certain types of problems. Which one would not apply for using restraints?

a. wandering
b. positioning problems
c. verbal abuse problems
d. falling problems
e. walking problems
Answer: c

149. What type of device would you call canes, crutches, and walkers?

a. orthotic
b. prosthetic
c. assistive
Answer: c

150. Which of the following would be considered a sign of impending death?

a. resident wanting ice cream
b. resident requesting to make a phone call
c. irregular breathing

d. rapid, weak, and irregular pulse
e. drop in respiration
f. c, d, and e would apply
Answer: f

151. How would a "clue" be defined?

a. symptoms as well as signs of infection that you can observe during your caring of a resident
b. something that the staff nurse tells you
c. something you have a "hunch" about
d. a symptom that the resident explains to you
Answer: a

152. When a gradual loss of minerals from the bones occur it usually makes the bones weak and brittle. What is this condition referred to as?

a. bursitis
b. rheumatism
c. osteoarthritis
d. osteoporosis
e. phlebitis
Answer: d

153. How would you define "continuous supportive care"?

a. temporary care in order to give relatives a break
b. care for the terminally ill only
c. care for children and infants only
d. care that is given on an "on going basis"
Answer: d

154. It is important to use the proper safety precautions when working with a resident's safety. Which of these would apply?

a. always lift under the resident's armpits
b. never lift without a "gait belt"
c. encourage residents to use bed rails, hand rails, grip rails
d. use quick motions

Answer: b

155. Mucous membranes, toenails, fingernails and hair would be considered extensions of which system?

a. reproductive
b. respiratory
c. circulatory
d. endocrine
e. integumentary

Answer: e

156. Which person would not be considered to be a part of the "nursing team"?

a. director of nursing
b. nurse assistant
c. director of staff development
d. physical therapist

Answer: c

157. Where would you locate the apical pulse?

a. in the second and third fingers

b. in the neck
c. at the wrist
d. below the left nipple
Answer: d

158. A sign of urinary retention is:

a. difficulty urinating
b. increased urinary output
c. swelling
d. decreased urinary output
e. a and d apply
Answer: e

159. Normal respirations at rest are between:

a. 25-35 per minute
b. 12-20 per minute
c. 18-24 per minute
d. 6-14 per minute
Answer: b

160. Which is not one of the parts of the chain of transmission of infection?

a. susceptible host
b. portal or route of exit
c. microorganisms
d. hand washing
Answer: d

161. Listed below is a heart rate that does not fall within the "normal range". Which one would apply?

a. 72
b. 64
c. 104
d. 84

Answer: d

162. The first place to gather information about a resident would be who?

a. their social worker
b. their physician
c. closest friend
d. the administrator
e. the resident

Answer: e

163. Hand washing is perhaps the most important thing to remember to do during your shift. What is not part of the hand washing technique?

a. applying soap
b. scraping nails on palms of your hands
c. drying thoroughly on clean paper towels
d. wiping your hands on your "clean uniform" is okay

Answer: d

164. Residents usually lose many things in a facility. Which ones would apply?

a. loss of privacy
b. loss of personal possessions

c. loss of physical ability/health
d. all of these apply
Answer: d

165. Long term care facilities have many names. Which ones would apply?

a. Nursing Home
b. Assisted living centers
c. rehabilitation centers
d. convalescent homes
e. all of these apply
Answer: e

166. Mindful care-giving means which of the following?

a. being intuitive and doing it "your way"
b. using your mind
c. knowing how to use the right and left brain parts of your mind
d. paying close attention to details, being observant as well as open
Answer: d

167. Sexual needs involve which of the below listed expressions?

a. emotional feelings only
b. only young people have these needs
c. only physical feelings
d. loving, caring feelings shared between people
Answer: d

168. If a hearing aid whistles you would check which of the following?

   a. to see if the ear mold is fitting properly
   b. see if the tubes and cords are connected properly
   c. to see if the battery contacts might be corroded
   d. just turn down the volume
   e. a, b, and c would apply

   Answer: e

169. There are several assistive devices i.e. walkers, crutches, and canes. There are basic guidelines for measuring assistive devices that are used in ambulation. Which would apply in the case of using a cane?

   a. cane should be at the level of trochanter with shoulders level, (not elevated or depressed when walking.)
   b. 20 degrees to 30 degrees flexion of the elbow upon movement
   c. cane should always have a metal tip on the end
   d. a and b apply

   Answer: d

170. When using crutches, which would apply?

   a. should be measured from axilla to the floor, then you would add 2" to 4"
   b. the hand grip level should be adjusted to allow 20 to 30 degrees flexion of elbow when moving forward
   c. you should be able to insert two or three fingers between the auxiliary pad on the crutch and the

axilla when the crutches are forwarded 4 to 6" out to the side.

d. all of the above apply

Answer: d

171. Listed below are some eating aids. Which ones apply?

a. sure grip glass holder
b. swivel utensils i.e. plastic handles
c. universal cuffs, suction bases, utensil holders
d. plate guard, special straw holders
e. horizontal palm self-handle utensil
f. extension utensils, non-slip pads
g. all of the above - know all of these

Answer: g

172. When a person is using a "walker", the walker should be at the height of the greater trochanter with approximately ______degrees flexion at the elbows when the walker is moved forward. Fill in the blank.

a. 20 degrees
b. 5 degrees
c. 45 degrees
d. 17 degrees

Answer: a

173. Which of the following would be considered to be "dressing and grooming" assistive devices?

a. rounded apical
b. built-up bursa
c. button aid
d. zipper pull

e. helping hand reacher
f. stocking aid
g. built-up handle toothbrush
h. c through g
Answer: h

174. There are three methods of taking temperature. Please match the three methods, the normal temperature for each type/method, and the time it takes to take these temperatures.

a. axillary (1) 99.6 - takes 5 minutes (reduce 1 deg.)
b. oral (2) 97.6 - takes 10 minutes (add 1 deg.)
c. Rectal (3) 98.6 - takes 3 minutes
Answer: b is (3), a is (2) and c is (1)

175. Name the three easy places to feel a pulse.

(1)
(2)
(3)

Answer:
side of neck (carotid area)
apical (apex of heart)
wrist (radial)

176. When would you use the axillary method for taking a temperature?

When the _________ or the ________ of the person can't be used for taking a temperature.

Answer: mouth or the anus (rectum)

177. If an individual has problems with their hands that may require occupational therapy intervention , please list at least 5 reasons that could require therapy.

Answer: painful hands - swollen hands - weakness stiff joints, un-coordination, can't hold spoons, tremors, hands too tight - difficult to clean

178. In doing Range of Motion exercises for the arm and the shoulder please give an example of how movement would be in flexion, extension, abduction, and adduction. What direction etc.?

Answer: Extension of the elbow you would straighten the arm and in the abduction of the arm you would raise the arm up and away from the body; in the adduction of the arm you would bring the arm down and toward the body and in the flexion you would bend the elbow and bring it toward the chest and back down to a table top level or more while holding your wrist with your other hand (if able to do so)

179. It is very important to do all Range Of Motion exercises slowly. What sequence would you follow (after identifying the starting joint) in the Range of Motion exercise for the "Shoulder Joint?"

Answer: first you would do flexion and extension - arm would go straight up and return (2) then abduction and adduction - arm would go out to the side and then return (3) horizontal abduction and adduction - arm would move in a lateral plane to opposite shoulder (4)

internal and external rotation - would be like a person directing traffic in a stop and go type of movements and finally, (5) hyperextension - this would be pointing your fingers behind your body keeping your elbow in a straight line.

180. There are at least (3) types of Range of Motion exercises. They are AROM, PROM, and AAROM. Please define each one of these and the moves.

Answer: AAROM is Active Assistant Range of Motion = a patient would have the assistance of another in order to complete a Range of Motion exercise
PROM is Passive Range of Motion = a patient is passive and the CNA, PT or OT would be doing the moving
AROM is Active Range of Motion = the patient is able to do the ROM's with no outside assistance

181. Please list at least 3 "feeding problems" that would require Occupational Therapy.

Answer: drooling problems, swallowing problems, and would not be able to hold eating utensils very well

182. If a resident's hearing aid is weak, list at least (2) things you would check for:

Answer: you would check to see if the battery was the correct size for their hearing air and also check to see if the volume control is in the right setting

183. There is a hearing aid called an ITE. What does this stand for?

____________ ____________ ____________

Answer: In the ear

184. Would you take out the hearing aid of a patient in the evening upon retiring or would you leave it in so they can hear whatever is going on around them?

Answer: You would take it out each evening and then put it back in the patient's ear in the morning

185. If you are removing a hearing aid from a patient what are two things that you normally check for or do?

Answer: you would check the ear mold for any wax and you would open the battery compartment

186. How often should a hearing aid battery be replaced?

Answer: every 2 to 3 weeks

187. In body alignment and positioning, it is very important to encourage AAROM whenever possible. What does this mean?

Answer: Active Assistant Range of Motion = the patient moves with assistance of another person to complete ROM's

188. If you are doing a hip and leg ROM (Abduction), describe how this would be done.

Answer: While on your back, your legs would be flat, straight. You would straighten your leg and then move away from the midline of the body.

189. Please describe what a pulse is and describe in detail how you would take a radial pulse.

Answer: A pulse is the beating of the heart that is sending blood through the arteries of the body. To take a radial pulse, you would take it at the wrist - radial artery and it may be counted while you are taking the temperature. You need a watch with a second hand. First of all, you would explain to the person that you are going to take their pulse. Be sure that you have washed your hands. Place the person's arm in a comfortable position. Find their pulse by putting the tips of your middle three fingers on the palm side of the person's wrist, in a line with their thumb next to the bone. Be sure that you NEVER use your thumb because your thumb has a pulse and you would feel that pulse. After you have found their pulse, press lightly, not too hard or you could stop the flow of their blood. Watch your second hand of your watch and start counting the beats you feel and count until the second hand has come back to the number on your watch when you started counting. Always count for <u>(1) one full minute,</u> making sure that you notice if their pulse beat is irregular, strong, weak, steady or unsteady. Be sure to record the number of beats you have counted and any irregular beats.

190. Please give 5 examples of joints that can rotate.

Answer: wrists, neck, hip, ankle and shoulder

191. Vital signs include at least (4) things. What are they?

Answer: respiratory rate, pulse rate, temperature, blood pressure

192. A pressure bulb with a control valve is part of a ______ and is used only when______?

Answer: cuff - taking someone's blood pressure

193. What is considered to be an abnormal diastolic blood pressure?

Answer: anything over 90

194. List the (4) things that you do when measuring a person's respiratory rate.

Answer:
(1) count their respiratory rate after their pulse rate,
(2) while keeping your fingers on the person's radial pulse, you would be watching the person's inspiration and expiration (making sure that you are not obvious about what you are watching because they could become self-conscious),
(3) you would count the respiratory rate for 1 minute just like you did their pulse rate and,
(4) you would record their respiratory rate and you would also make sure that you would report anything out of the ordinary to the Charge Nurse

195. When you are filling the Companion 1000 unit from the stationary please list at least (ONE) CAUTION

pertaining to the connectors before filling, and at least (ONE) WARNING PERTAINING TO THE Companion 1000.

Answer: Before you fill the Companion 1000 with oxygen it is important to make sure that all of the connectors are clean and dry in order to avoid any malfunction due to freezing. A WARNING when filling is: if liquid oxygen should happen to leak when the portable is disengaged, proceed to re-engage and disengage the unit. This will help to dislodge any ice or other obstruction. If liquid leakage is still present, call maintenance IMMEDIATELY. DO NOT WAIT

196. Is the Endocrine System the system that is used by most Long Term Care Facilities when indoctrinating new CNA's? Yes or No.

Answer: No

197. Is it true that cataracts appear in the right eye first? Yes or No.

Answer: No

198. Does NPO stand for Never Push Occupant? Yes or No

Answer: No

199. What does NPO stand for?

Answer: Nothing by Mouth

200. What would be the first step in a bladder retraining program?

Answer: You would check to see is the resident can participate on their own

CHAPTER SIX
MOBILITY, RESPIRATORY, CIRCULATORY, HYGIENE, and BOWEL AND BLADDER ELIMINATION NEEDS

~ ~ ~ ~ ~ ~

WHAT YOU NEED TO KNOW ABOUT
INSULIN REACTIONS and TERMINOLOGY

1. An insulin reaction occurs when there is too much ______ and too little ________ in the blood.

   Too much insulin and too little sugar

2. Hypoglycemia is the medical term for ____ _____ ____.

   Low Blood sugar

3. There are several signs and symptoms of an Insulin Reaction. Symptoms develop rapidly – within 15 minutes to one hour – and vary with the individual. Name at least thirteen symptoms that could possible occur with an Insulin Reaction.

   dulness
   headache
   irritability
   crying
   shaking
   sweating
   lightheadedness
   hunger
   change in mood or behavior
   numbness of lips or tongue

pale skin
weakness
moist skin

4. If Insulin Reaction is not treated properly, these above symptoms may progress to what?

   confusion
   unconsciousness
   loss of coordination
   slurred speech
   dizziness

5. An Insulin Reaction at night may cause two things. What are they?

   excessive dreaming or sweating
   morning headache

6. When a resident's fingernail beds are bluish in color, this indicates the resident is not getting enough ________.

   oxygen

7. The main reason most elderly people become incontinent of urine is because the ________ related to urination become weak.

   muscles

8. When a resident dies, when should the nurse assistant begin postmortem care?

   after death has been pronounced

9. What is the most important thing a nurse assistant should do to increase both the respiratory and the circulatory functions of a resident who is in a coma?

   make sure they change the position of the resident every two hours

10. How often should the nurse assistant release a mitt restraint a resident has been wearing in order to exercise and massage the resident's hand?

    every two hours

11. If a resident wants to use a bedpan, the nurse assistant should place the resident on the bedpan in which position? Sitting or reclining position?

    sitting position

12. The most important thing the nurse assistant needs to do when working with a resident who is ambulated is to _______.

    report to the nurse what the response was

13. If a resident has some questions she would like to ask her doctor but can't seem to remember all of them, what is the best thing the nurse assistant can do to help her remember?

    Offer her some paper and a pen or pencil to write down the questions

14. If a nurse assistant notices bright red mucus from coming from a resident's mouth who appears to have difficulty breathing, this should be reported to the nurse immediately because it

could be an indication that the resident could have ______ _______ _______.

chronic respiratory disease

15. If a resident is obese, in what position would they have the most trouble breathing?

    supine position (flat on their back)

16. It is very important for the nurse assistant to do what with the wheelchair, when moving a resident from the bed to the wheelchair?

    lock the wheels on the wheelchair before moving the resident

17. If a resident who is in a wheelchair asks the nurse assistant to go to the bathroom, and they voided 20 minutes ago, what should the nurse assistant do?

    take the resident to the bathroom and place them on the toilet as they may have to go again

18. If the nurse assistant is going to lift a resident, what is the best and safest position to be in?

    stand with feet wide apart and one foot placed forward

19. True or False. If a person drinks an excessive amount of fluids this will stretch the bladder and they would have the urge to urinate before the bladder becomes full or stretched.

    True

20. True or False. A person will gain weight when their urine output is less than the fluid intake.

    True

21. What should the nurse assistant do to help prevent skin breakdown when the resident is incontinent of loose stools, and is also impaired mentally?

    Check the rectal area frequently for any soiling

22. What would the nurse assistant use as the safest method to move an obese paralyzed resident to a chair?

    They would use a Hoyer Lift

23. If a Doctor orders a resident to wear elastic stockings, the nurse assistant should put them on the resident at what time of day? Just before bedtime or first thing in the a.m.?

    Elastic stockings should be put on before the resident gets out of their bed in the morning

24. Define a transfer belt.

    It is a device that is used to transfer a resident from a chair to a bed.

25. What is the 'Fowler's position' used for?

    To relieve those who have difficulty breathing caused by heart disease, pulmonary disease, obesity and other causes.

26. Define in detail what the Fowler's position is.

The head, neck and trunk of the resident are raised by elevating the head of the bed 45 degrees to the Fowler's position or up to 90 degrees which is referred to as the high Fowler's position. The semi Fowler position is when the resident is raised up only 45 degrees (halfway). This position is reached by placing pillows under the back, neck and head OR by elevating the head of the bed.

27. When a nurse assistant signs a signature and or initial to the turning schedule for a resident who is on bed rest, and is on a turning, positioning schedule every two hours, what does it mean when the nurse assistant signs the schedule?

    It means the resident was turned at the time it was signed and/or initialed.

28. Sometimes a resident will mention things that they are sorry they did. One lady was telling a nurse assistant she felt sad because she didn't give her children enough attention when they were growing up. What should the nurse assistant do and why?

    The nurse assistant could say something like, "Oh, so you feel you were neglecting your children?" A remark like this may open up levels of communication whereby they can talk about their feelings of remorse and some guilt they've held in for years that was never resolved in their mind.

29. What should the nurse assistant do when ambulating a resident with a urinary catheter?

    They should make sure they hold the bag below the level of the bladder.

30. Give an example of a resident having an inability to accept their limitations.

    When a resident insists on doing something that they can not possibly do (i.e. get up out of a wheelchair when they can't walk).

31. When a resident is getting oxygen through a nasal cannula, why is it important not to remove the cannula every few hours for 15 minute intervals?

    You should never remove oxygen, except when cleaning the nose and openings promptly, as this would cause skin to breakdown.

32. If a resident has a Foley catheter and it is placed on the wheelchair, where should the nurse assistant should place the drainage bag?

    it should be hooked on the side of the wheelchair below the bladder

33. What is the first thing the nurse assistant should tell a resident who is being placed on oxygen therapy?

    Tell the resident they can not smoke near oxygen, and can not have any petroleum jelly in the room.

34. A resident is showing signs of sadness and loss of appetite, and is in pain a great deal of the time. She can not do simple things for herself. Would this be a sign she is depressed?

    Yes

35. What are some of the things the nurse assistant should do when changing a condom catheter OR (sometimes referred to as an external catheter?)

Hang the drainage bag on the bed frame, make sure the tubing from the catheter does not get caught under the resident's legs, and roll the condom up the shaft of the penis

36. When you are transporting a resident in a wheelchair onto an elevator, what is the proper procedure when entering the elevator?

You would always turn the wheelchair around and enter the elevator with the large wheels first

37. When would hugging be appropriate by the nurse assistant ?

When a resident seems to be confused. Hugs are a form of communication, and they communicate a caring which sometimes eliminates fear.

38. What should a nurse assistant do when providing mouth care for a resident who is unconscious?

It is important to explain what you are going to do, and why you are going to do it.

39. Matted hair is very common for people who are on what?

Complete bed rest.

40. List three things the Nurse Assistant should do when applying wrist restraints.

(1) Tie the straps to the bed frame.
(2) Make sure a call bell is within reach.
(3) Be sure and pad the wrists with something soft.

41. There is one things the Nurse Assistant should never do when applying wrist restraints. What is it?

Never use a double knot when securing the straps.

42. When a resident is admitted to a nursing home, and he/she begins to cry when their family leaves, what could be one of the reasons for their crying?

Anxiety

43. Why would the Nurse Assistant have to use restraints?

In order to protect the resident from harming themselves.

44. How often should a resident be turned in order to reduce pressure?

Approximately every two hours

45. When a resident is dying and they cries frequently and is sad, what should the nurse assistant do?

Try to stay with the resident as much as possible.

46. If a resident wakes up and complains of being short of breath, what should the nurse assistant do?

    Raise the head of their bed.

47. A bedsore is sometimes referred to as a decubitus ulcer. What is sometimes used to prevent bedsores?

    An egg crate mattress.

48. True or False. A Draw Sheet is one piece of linen that is least likely to be reused for the same resident?

    True

49. Why are ROM (Range of Motion) exercises important?

    They help to keep the joints moving.

50. True or False. A low calorie, low salt diet is sometimes ordered by the Dr. if the resident is overweight and retains fluid in their legs and ankles.

    True

Daily Intake and Output Record

Resident Name: Date:

Shift

7 a.m. – 3 p.m. Fluid Intake | 7 - 3 Fluid Output | Comments

Time	Amount	Type	Time	Amount	Type	
8:15	135	Juice				
9:00	125		Water	9:00	310	Urine
1:00	290	Coffee	11:00	210	Urine	
3:00	320	Water	1:30	100	Urine	
			2:45	50	Vomitus	
TOTAL:			TOTAL:			

51. A resident is on I & O. On the above I & O, what is the total fluid intake for the 7 a.m. to 3 p.m. shift?

    870 cc (ml)

52. On the above I & O, what would be the total output during the 7 a.m. - 3 p.m. shift?

    Total urine output is 620 + the vomitus (50) would be a total output of 670 cc.

53. What is the normal range for an oral temperature?

    Between 97.6° and 99.6°

54. After the nurse assistant has washed her hands, the water faucet should be turned off with what?

    A clean dry paper towel.

55. What is the normal range for respirations?

14 to 20 breaths per minute

56. What would be the 1st thing the nurse assistant would do after the doctor ordered 1,100 cc (ml) of fluid restriction per day?

Place a sign at the bedside that reads, "Restrict Fluids."

57. What are the benefits of flotation pads and/or gel cushions?

They help to spread the body weight.

58. What is the proper way of making a bed in order to prevent bedsores?

The bottom sheet should be pulled very tight.

59. True or False. If a resident has had a stroke, would they be considered a high risk for getting decubitus ulcers?

True

60. True or False. 90/60 mm Hg would be considered normal in the elderly.

False

61. When doing Range of Motion exercises, what would opening a fist be referred to as?

An Extension

62. If a resident is on bed rest, they are a high risk for developing what?

Decubitus ulcers (bed sores)

63. What is the most important thing the Nurse Assistant should do when taking a rectal temperature with a glass thermometer?

They should NEVER let go of the thermometer when it is in the resident.

64. True or False. When feeding a resident, who has recently had a stroke and has right-sided weakness, one of the things the Nurse Assistant should never do is to place soft food on the weak side of the mouth.

True

65. Which of the following would be the correct time of day when the resident's body temperature is at it's lowest?

1. 5 a.m.
2. 10 a.m.
3. 3 p.m.
4. 7:30 p.m.

Answer: (a) 5 a.m.

66. If a resident has had an iced drink, how long should the Nurse Assistant wait before taking an oral temperature?

15 minutes

67. When putting a dress on a resident who has weakness in her left side, what is the first thing the Nurse Assistant should remember?

Put the resident's left arm through the left sleeve first.

68. What does the radial pulse rate measure?

The function of the heart.

69. What two pieces of equipment does the Nurse Assistant need in order to take a person's blood pressure?

Stethoscope and a sphygmomanometer.

70. Yes or No. Can a decubitus ulcer can be caused by pressure?

Yes

71. With a standing scale, name at least three things that the Nurse Assistant should do.

(1) Make sure to balance the scales before taking the weight.
(2) Make sure the resident stands in the middle of the scale.
(3) Write down the weight as soon as it is taken.

72. There is a proper way of removing dirty linens from an occupied bed? How should the Nurse Assistant do this?

Roll the linens into itself. Never shake the linens.

73. Why is hand washing so important?

It prevents spreading of infection in long term care facilities,

and it is the best thing the Nurse Assistant can do for themselves as well in order not to spread microorganisms.

74. Why is it important to know what the height of a new resident who was just admitted into a care facility?

To determine what the best weight should be for the resident.

75. Is it okay for the Nurse Assistant to use a resident's roommate's comb and brush if it looks clean?

NO. NEVER!

76. Would anxiety be considered an example of objective data?

NO

77. True or False. In order to clean a glass thermometer after using it, the Nurse Assistant should wash it with soap and cool water because soap and friction helps to loosen the microorganisms and dirt. Using cool water douses the thermometer, preventing it from breaking from using hot water

True

78. How long does it take for the mouth to recover from drinking an iced drink and return to the resident's normal body temperature?

15 minutes

79. Should a fire occur, and a fire extinguisher is available, should the Nurse Assistant point the hose to extinguish the fire?

The hose should be pointed at the base of the fire.

80. Bed making is very important in a care facility. What would be the most important objective in making a bed for a resident?

To make the resident as comfortable as possible.

81. Can a class A fire extinguisher put out a fire in a storage closet?

NO, because most storage closets house flammable liquids and cleaners, thus causing the fire to spread if it were used. Also, a class A fire extinguisher contains water; and water should not be used in a kitchen or on any electrical fire because water would conduct electricity and grease can splatter.

82. Many times a resident has lost their spouse and grieves often. When they cry, what should the Nurse Assistant do?

Stay with the resident while they are crying as this shows concern, caring, and acceptance. It also provides emotional support for the resident. You DON'T want to do anything that would deny how the resident feels (i.e. changing the subject.)

83. If a resident begins vomiting in bed, it's important for the Nurse Assistant to place the resident's head in the proper, safe position? What would that be?

Hold their head to the side, as this would help to prevent the resident from choking and help to drain the mouth.

84. What is a contracture?

A muscle that is drawn or shortened.

85. What causes contractures?

Lying in bed too long.

86. What is dysphagia?

Difficulty swallowing.

87. What is aphasia?

Defective or absent language ability.

88. What is dementia?

It is a severe state of cognitive impairment characterized by memory loss, difficulty with abstract thinking, and disorientation.

89. What is the definition of body mechanics?

It is using the body properly to prevent injury when lifting, moving, and bending.

90. Define continence.

It is the control of the bowel function and control of the bladder.

91. Define cyanosis.

It is the blue color of any part of the body due to lack of oxygen.

92. What is systolic pressure?

It is the top number of the blood pressure that reflects pressure in vessels when the heart is beating.

93. What is Fowler's position?

Sitting upright.

94. What is ileostomy?

It is a surgical opening of the ileum (small intestine) on the surface of the abdomen, where fecal contents are collected in an external appliance.

95. What is the definition of pathologic?

It is disease-causing pathology.

96. Define palpate.

Use of touch to assess.

97. Define ombudsman.

It is a resident representative who investigates reported complaints and helps to achieve agreement between parties (i.e. resident/family and staff)

98. Define Nurse Assistant.

    A trained member of the health care team who provides the majority of hands-on resident care.

99. What does oral mean?

    In the mouth.

100. Define subjective observations.

    Individual guesses or hunches based on objective information.

101. What is dyspnea?

    Difficulty breathing.

102. Define emesis.

    It is vomit.

103. What are hemorrhoids?

    Enlarged blood vessels at the anus that look like flat or swollen tags of skin.

104. Define mindfulness.

    It is interacting with others by paying attention to details, looking at situations openly, and being observant and flexible

105. What does nonpathologic mean?

It is not diesease-causing.

106. What are objective observations?

They are undisputable facts.

107. Define orientation.

It is the ability to accurately identify a person, place, and time. It is also to be shown something new (i.e. a new procedure, job, etc.)

108. Define perineal care.

It is cleansing of the perineum (the area between the thighs, the external genitals and anus).

109. Sterile means.....

Free of all germs.

110. Define lubricant.

A slippery substance such as petroleum jelly, which facilitates passage of instruments into body orifices.

111. You would NOT want to have petroleum jelly near what?

Oxygen equipment in use.

112. List two functions of the dietary division.

To provide food that is clean/safe/appealing, and to also administer diets that have to be modified.

Chapter Seven

Important Skills You Should Know As A Care Giver

Perhaps the ***most important skill*** I learned when studying to become a Nurse Assistant was the correct way to wash your hands. Rule number one. Don't wear a lot of bracelets, and you may consider not wearing a wrist watch either. Most long term care facilities have wall clocks in most areas if you need to see what time it is. Keep your watch in a pocket, and when you need to use it (i.e. when taking vital signs), you can put it back in your pocket and not worry about removing it every time you wash your hands— which is frequently.

The correct way to wash your hands is:

- Be sure to remove any jewelry, watches; and if you are wearing long sleeves, roll those up.
- Make sure the water is an acceptable temperature.
- Wet your hands and include your wrists as well.
- From the soap dispenser, apply adequate soap and rub your hands in a circular motion for approx. 8-10 seconds, making sure you are creating some friction.
- Lace your fingers together and slide them back and forth.
- Make sure your palm is soapy, and with your right hand, take your fingernails and scratch your left palm, using all of your five fingernails as though you had an itch on your palm. This helps to clean underneath your nails. Repeat the same procedure with your left hand, scratching your right palm.
- You want to now rinse your hands, making sure the water is warm; and be sure to keep your arms downward, wrists and hands downward as you rinse off the soap. This will allow the water to run from the wrist downward to the fingers rinsing the entire hands.

- Don't turn off the water yet, even though you are ready to dry your hands.
- With a clean paper towel, begin to dry your hands starting with wrists, moving downward as you dry your fingers.
- With the paper towel that you used to dry your fingers, turn off the water.
- Discard paper towel.

NOTE: At the long term care facility where my training was held, the Instructor suggested taking another paper towel before leaving the restroom or area where you washed your hands, and use it to open the door. Why? People carry germs on their hands and door knobs become one of the filthiest places where germs accumulate. Just use a clean towel to open the door and then when you leave that area, discard the paper towel you used to open the door into the nearest trash container.

Preparation For The Body After Death

- Always treat the body with utmost respect.
- If that resident shared a room with another resident, and that resident is cognizant of their surroundings, it is very important to make sure that the roommate is not in the room when you are preparing the body after death. This is very upsetting to the roommate.
- Pull all curtains for privacy, and be sure and close the door completely.
- If the resident had any tubes, dressings, etc., you want to remove those.
- Place the body in a supine (flat) position, with the limbs straight, and place one pillow under their head. This prevents their face and neck from becoming discolored.
- Be sure to put in their dentures.

- Prepare the body by washing it, just like you would if you were giving them a bed bath, and put fresh dressing over any wounds.
- Fix their hair (comb it.)
- Be sure and cover the perineal area with a pad, so that it can absorb drainage and then put a clean gown on the body.

NOTE: The following are skills you should be prepared to know before becoming a nurse assistant. If you do NOT now how to perform these skills be sure and ask your Instructor to go over these with you before you take your exam. I am just listing these and not describing them step by step.

Know how to:

- move a resident from supine position to a sitting position
- move a resident to the side of the bed using the drawsheet
- move to the side of the bed when a resident is unable to help
- move the resident up in bed when they can help
- move the resident up in bed when they can't help you
- move to the side of the bed when a resident can help
- turn a resident from supine to side lying for personal care
- put on gloves properly
- remove gloves properly
- put on a gown properly
- remove the gown properly
- put on a mask and how to remove the mask
- give a complete bed bath
- perform perineal care for female and male residents
- position a resident in a chair correctly
- give a tub bath
- give a shower
- give a whirlpool bath
- shampoo and condition the resident's hair

- make an unoccupied bed
- make an occupied bed
- undress a dependent resident
- help the resident use the bedpan
- help the resident use the urinal
- help the residents eat
- use a portable commode
- take an oral temperature
- take blood pressure
- take respiratory rate
- take a radial pulse
- take an apical pulse
- take an axillary temperature
- take a rectal temperature
- take an oral temperature
- collect a urinalysis specimen
- collect a sputum specimen
- perform the Heimlich Maneuver
- do Range of Motion Exercises
- help the resident use a portable commode
- walk properly with the resident using the guard belt
- do the stand pivot transfer
- move a resident with a mechanical lift
- transfer a resident from a chair to the bed or the toilet
- properly do the assisted transfer with an assistive device
- to do the Fowler's Position
- move a resident up in a chair
- return a resident to bed using a mechanical lift
- to properly position a resident on his or her back
- care for dentures, brush and floss
- shave resident's underarms, legs, male resident's face
- perform mouth care for comatose residents
- trim facial hair

- care for fingernails and toenails
- dress a dependent resident
- measure weight and height using an upright scale
- collect a urinalysis specimen
- collect a clean catch urinalysis specimen
- collect a stool specimen
- test urine for sugars, acetone, ketones, and glucose

NOTE: It is very important to know all aspects of oxygen equipment, changing equipment, and all other equipment that is used in the resident's room.

NEVER SMOKE IN AN AREA WHERE THERE IS OXYGEN EQUIPMENT. NEVER HAVE ANY PETROLEUM JELLY NEAR OXYGEN.

Items Needed For Various Personal Care

192. What items would you need when providing care of the toenails?

2 towels
soap
wash cloth
orangewood stick
shoes and socks
lotion
fill the wash basin half full with warm water

193. What items would you need when providing care of the fingernails?

towel
wash cloth
soap
orangewood stick
lotion
nail clippers
nail file or emery board

194. What items would you need to make an occupied bed?

2 sheets (full)
draw sheet
blanket and spread
pillowcases

195. What items would you need to make an unoccupied bed?

2 full sheets
blanket and spread
draw sheet (if needed)
pillowcases

196. What items would you need when dressing a dependent resident?

Clothes to wear
undergarments
plastic-covered pad
stockings, socks, shoes
any accessories resident wants to wear (jewelry, tie, etc.)

197. What items would you need when undressing a dependent resident?

The clothes they wear after undressing

198. What items would you need to shave a male resident's face?

wash cloth
mirror
gloves
razor
shaving cream
cologne if they use it
towel
plastic bag
wash basin half filled with warm water

199. When giving a complete bed bath list the items you would need.

basin half full of warm water
2 wash cloths
towels
bedpan
gloves
soap
lotion
plastic trash bag
plastic covered pad and/or protective covering
bath blanket

200. List four types of communication.

Touch
listening
verbal communication
nonverbal communication

201. Why is communication important with the residents?

It helps to improve each resident's quality of life, makes your job easier and also more enjoyable, and everyone likes to know they are being heard.

202. List five examples of nonverbal communication.

Eye contact
body language
touch
sitting down to talk
facial expressions

203. If a resident has hearing loss what can you do to help improve communication with them?

Point to objects
face the resident when you are talking with them

Define The Following Words

body Mechanics	=	taking care to insure correct body position in order to prevent any injury to you and the resident
ergonomics	=	relationships between workers and their jobs
Material Safety Data Sheets	=	describes chemical contents, fire hazards and first aid (MSDS)

mindful	=	assessing a situation and paying attention to details
common-sense	=	making sure you know your resident's needs Rules
nutrition	=	balanced supply of food
chemotherapy	=	a form of cancer treatment that uses drugs
chronic	=	process of long duration
radiation	=	a form of cancer treatment that uses X-rays

204. Define in detail what a Long Term Care Facility is.

It can be a rehab center, nursing home, or residential care facility that provides special services to people with special needs that can't be given in the person's home or should not be given in the persons home.

205. Federal Rules and Regulations state that a Long Term Care Facility must provide what services?

social
nursing
dietary
administrative
pharmacy
dental
specialized
physician

206. What should you know about a walking cane?

- **Physical therapy evaluates the size and length of the cane, and the cane is to be placed on affected side no further than 1 step's length forward.**
- **Use a gait belt if SBA (Stand by assist) is necessary (CNA to stand on *unaffected* side.)**

207. What do you know about Bowel and Bladder Program?

The purpose is to help the resident regain as much control over bowel or urinary function as possible. What you to for people on a bowel and bladder program is follow a regular schedule of toileting everyday, 24 hours a day. Encourag the resident to go to the bathroom on a regular schedule, or assist the resident with limited mobility to the bathroom, or commode at regular intervals.
Also, it is very important to first keep a record of the resident's voiding pattern, including recording time of voiding, AMT voided, fluid voided, fluid intact, and awareness of needing to void.

208. What do you know about walking with crutches?

The physical therapy dept should evaluate the height of crutches. Your body should never be further forward than the crutches. Use gait belt if resident needs stand by assistance; or better place one foot forward, ("one steps's worth") forward only. The resident should then move up to the crutches. The resident should not move their body past the crutches ever. The steps should then be repeated.

209. What does Stand By Assistance mean?

It means a person can walk and sit alone, no gait belt required. (an independent person.)

210. What does CGA stand for?

Contact Guard Assistance. You want to have initial contact, touching but not holding them up.

211. What does MIN stand for?

Minimum assistance - will help a little bit.

212. What does MOD stand for?

Moderate assistance.

213. What does MAX stand for?

Maximum assist - they can bear weight, they are not totally dependent.

214. What does T stand for?

Total assist - they cannot do anything, require total transfers

215. If a resident is using a walker, what would the procedure be?

Resident needs to move walker one steps' worth forward only. They then need to step forward to the walker. Then repeat.

216. What makes up the endocrine system?

1. **Glands - release hormones used in another part of body**
2. **Endocrine Glands - pancreas - thyroid, regulates metabolism; total of all body processes.**
3. **Metabolic Processes - build up, repair tissue after injury or changing food into fat that can be stored for later use; breaking down, using stored fat for energy.**

INSULIN

Insulin eats up sugar in your body.

Changes:	**Effect**:
Decrease in insulin production during stressful situations	Fatigue during stress
Decrease in ability of body to use insulin	Usually no symptoms

Diabetes Mellitus (decrease in insulin produced by pancreas):

- Most severe in kids - young adults
- Elderly, due to being over weight usually no symptoms but increase in level of sugar

Complications:
Associated with thickening of blood vessels that inhibit blood flow to vital organs causes
decrease in vision

- kidney failure
- heart attack
- stroke

Foot Care

- treat cut not healing due to decrease in circulation
- observe feet daily- look for cuts and redness
- dry between toes carefully
- wear well fitting shoes
- wear socks with shoes
- report to charge nurse if resident needs to have toes nails cut or fingernails cut

Monitoring control of Diabetes

- blood tests
- test urine
- 2nd voided specimen

List some signs of circulatory problems, and what is considered a normal blood pressure

- Normal blood pressure is 120/80
- Signs of circulatory problems are:
  1. High blood pressure
  2. Difficulty breathing during strenuous activity
  3. Abnormal heat rhythm (arrhythmic):
     a. Tachycardia ↑ Pulse > 100
     b. Bradycardia ↓ Pulse 50s
  4. Cool skin temperature.
  5. Reddish, mottled, bluish (waxy pale) look especially legs (arterial).
  6. Swelling (edema) feet and lower legs (venous decrease in circulation).

Assist - ℞ Increased in Blood Pressure

1. Reduce salt intake - control weight - makes heart pump harder
2. Use of medications to lower or control.

Report BP reading

Breathing

Meds - may help heart beat to become stronger and more regular - Assist By

Changing resident's position after 1-2 hours

Encourage to take daily walks and participate in exercise program

Avoid activity that interferes with circulation:

1. Crossing legs
2. Wearing restrictive clothing (avoid girdles and garters).
3. Smoking cigarettes, as it narrows blood vessels.
4. Encourage resident to wiggle toes, make circles with ankles.
5. Keep skin dry, clean and apply lotion as it improves their circulation.
6. Provide safe environment in order to prevent injury.

Major Complications:

Skin Breakdown - Assist Resident with swelling

- Sit with legs up on foot stool, or lie on bed with legs stretched out, 1-2 hours three times a day.
- Encourage resident to exercise and walk.
- Make sure shoes are not too tight.
- Wear support stockings and put them on while lying down. Be sure to take them off at night.

Things To Know About Abnormal Heart Rhythm:

Take Apical Pulse

have resident lie down
place stethoscope below nipple
count 2 minutes
you will hear two sounds:
lubb - dubb

Lubb - valves are closing between upper and lower chambers of the heart

Dubb - sound of valves closing after heart has pumped blood out of body

Note: rate and rhythm below 60 - above 100

Assist with Poor Circulation

Can lead to skin breakdown, infection, and loss of limb

Assess Feet:

temperature
color of skin
color of nailbeds: blanching
pulse in lower extremities
observe for reddened area, cracks between toes

Support Stockings:

ordered for resident with poor venous circulation
provide equal pressure from toes to knee
help blood flow up to veins in legs and back to heart

Purpose - Ted Hose

- Increase in venous return from legs and prevent pooling of blood edema of lower legs

Note: If resident has poor arterial and venous circulation, and Ted Hose is not ordered, there could be a decrease in arterial circulation.

Respiratory System Information

Respiration 16-24 breaths per minute
If it is into the 30s, there would be a concern
Respiratory rate 12-30 a minute
Cells need oxygen to function and live.

System consists of:

nose
trachea
right and left lung
bronchus
bronchioles
alveoli

Breathing

Cells need oxygen to function and to live

Changes	Effect
chest wall and lung more rigid lungs;	not as much room in the More difficult to take
decrease in number of air sacks	Have to breathe faster to get enough oxygen in and carbon dioxide out during exercise or stress; exhaling more difficult.

Practical Side

Assess Breathing Pattern In Older People = Rhythm

Respiration increases during moderate to strenuous exercise
observe visual respiratory rate
observe changes in rate or dyspnea (difficulty in breathing)
during A-D-L's (Activity of daily living)
report abnormal rate

Signs of Problems

Chronic Examples:

- increase in respiratory rate
- noisy respiration
- complains of shortness of breath
- skin color pale or bluish grey

Assist With Acute (short term i.e pneumonia, flu and/or colds)

- have resident sit or lie down with HOB (Head of Bed) upward - NOT FLAT
- encourage resident to relax and breathe slowly
- get the nurse

Assist With Chronic —

- take 4-5 deep breaths several times a day
- fill lungs with air, chest wall more flexible
- rest between ADL's
- encourage resident to breathe slowly and deeply while ambulatory (moving about, walking), and a minute during longer walks

Assisting With Residents Who Eat Poorly and Information You Need To Know

- make sure the dietician is aware of any likes and dislikes of the resident
- offer assistance frequently when resident is eating
- note things that discourage eating
- note if they have difficulty bring food to their mouth, chewing, swallowing, etc.
- discuss if they are depressed
- remember they may benefit from special eating utensils

Things Taught by OT (Occupational Therapy) Pertaining to Assisting Residents to Eat

- prepare food; cut it up and/or mush it
- DO NOT RUSH
- allow resident to feed themselves to the extent possible
- offer variety - not too hot
- use spoon and fork only ½ full
- make sure the resident chews and swallows each bite
- offer liquids to moisten food
- wash face after eating

Common Causes of Difficulty Swallowing

- strokes
- Parkinson's Disease
- M.S.

Progressive Diseases Affecting Nervous System Evaluated by Speech Pathologist

Result

- become malnourished
- aspiration pneumonia

Assist By

- getting the resident in an upright position
- give small bites of food
- small sips of water to moisten food
- be prepared to perform Heimlich Maneuver

Basic Food Groups

- milk - dairy products
- meat - fish- poultry
- fruits - vegetables
- grains

Results of Poor Eating

- general weakness
- inability to fight infection
- weight loss and/or weight gain

Food Supplements

- minerals and vitamins
- formulas
- supplemental feedings

Information on Exercise

- Reasons for exercising:
  vital part of life, it improves what we may be able to do

Benefits	Prevents
increase in muscle strength	Muscle weakness
maintain joint mobility	Contractures (when a joint freezes in a position)
improve coordination	Falls
improve self-image	Anxiety and depression
maintain or reduce weight	Obesity

Types of Exercises

- Walking : encourage those who can
  Assist those who can't
- Range of Motion: move joints to fullest ability
  a. Passive - do it for them
  b. Active - they can do it

Assistance With Movement

Why change position?

- helps use muscles
- move joints
- avoid pressure on only a few areas of the body

Principles In Movement

- Whenever possible, roll or slide instead of lifting resident
- move toward, rather than away; roll like a log

Assist From Bed To Chair

- lock wheelchair
- put foot rests, out of the way
- place chair at a 45 degree angle
- place on strong side
- stand on resident's weak side
- use Gait Belt
- make sure hips are in back of chair (support weak arm at elbow)
- make sure resident can reach signal cord
- support legs

CHANGE POSITION AFTER 2 HOURS.
SHIFT FREQUENTLY!

Reasons Residents May Not Exercise

- fear of hurting
- feelings of hopelessness
- not knowing if exercise will help them

How You Can Help The Resident To Exercise

- be enthusiastic and positive
- explain why it is important
- demonstrate / return
- demonstrate with resident ROM - don't rotate joint
- do flexion
- rub any area of the body that you are going to do ROM on in order to help get the circulation going
- be sure to support the area you are working on

The Three Reasons You Do NOT Cut Finger/Toenails

- resident is on blood thinners
- resident has circulatory problems
- diabetic - their wounds do not heal well

Information About a Graduate

Hang your Foley Bag on the part of the bed frame that moves. NEVER pick up the Graduate to measure it. Put it on a level surface and measure in cc's. 32 ozs - 950 cc

NEVER PUT A LEG BAG ON WHEN LYING DOWN OR AT NIGHT WHEN SLEEPING

NOTE: IF THE RESIDENT HAS A URINE INFECTION THE URINE MAY SMELL BAD, BE BROWN, CLOUDY AND BLOODY. THEY MAY HAVE A TEMPERATURE, BURNING SENSATION WHILE URINATING AND HAVE TO URINATE EVERY ½ HOUR OR SO.

Information About the Heart and Circulation

The heart is a muscle with 4 chambers and it pumps blood. The heart and blood vessels make up the circulatory system. The location of the heart is underneath ribs and between the two lungs. The largest part of the heart is the left side. It has the Right and Left Atrium and the Right and Left Ventricle. The body returns unoxygenated blood to the Right Atrium to the Aorta.

The Aorta shoots the blood back to the body and branches off to the upper and lower parts of the body. It connects with the smaller vessels, carries oxygenated blood to every organ and cell in the body.

NEVER TALK TO A RESIDENT AS IF THEY WERE A TWO YEAR OLD. EXPLAIN EVERYTHING YOU ARE GOING TO DO. CALL THEM MR. OR MRS. OR MS. SEE IF A RESIDENT CAN WRITE. COMMUNICATION IS VERY IMPORTANT.

Speech and Communications

Aphasia is difficulty understanding communication.
Assist residents who don't understand by doing the following:

- checking care plan
- always approach them with a calm, reassuring manner
- they may understand written communication
- point to objects and use gestures
- even if they can't understand spoken words, they can understand by written communication, pointing to objects, etc
- be patient, use a gentle loving touch often
- speak slowly - use simple sentences

Information About Eyes and Ears

Common Diseases:

- cataracts - general blurring of vision
- glaucoma - (increased pressure in the eye) - blurring of vision, rainbows around light - inability to see out of corners of eyes
- Macular Degeneration - difficult to treat - has peripheral (side) vision blurring of vision (what looks at directly)

Assisting Residents With Visual Problems

- know type of problem
- identify yourself
- stand where they can see you
- place objects where residents can see you
- make sure area is well lighted - turn on all lights
- keep all furnishings in same area as that becomes familiar to them
- think about activities that the resident may enjoy
- assist in ambulation - give control of movement and support
- use clock to explain the food i.e. = the clock is the plate, at exactly 6:00 o'clock the big hand is where the applesauce is and the little hand is where the meat is, etc.

Dangers You Should Report

- sudden decrease in vision
- rainbows around light
- pain in the resident's eyes- report within 24 hours
- redness in or around the eye and watch for any draining around the eye or any color grey/yellow matted crust around the eyes
- any sudden inability to recognize your face, or locate any familiar objects or not able to distinguish color

Note: With cataract glaucoma, be sure to know all definitions and how to help the residents out with eye care.

ALWAYS WEAR GLOVES - take a warm wash cloth to a matted eye and be gentle as you clean it.

Information About The Ears

- Wax is a lubricating system.
- Let nurses know about and ears that are stopped-up.
- With a loss of hearing, residents can't hear consonants s, t, c, & x, and they may become fearful, anxious, withdrawn and avoid friends and social events.
- The middle ear has three (3) bones.

Signs Of Ear Infections

- temperature
- when resident move about they lose sense of balance - feel dizzy
- sometimes when resident sits up they vomit
- with an increase of temperature they become nauseous

BE SURE AND TELL THE NURSE OF ALL SYMPTOMS

Assisting Residents With Ear Problems

- inform your nurse
- be at eye level and be sure and face the resident
- speak clearly and directly to the resident and drop your voice as deeply as possible
- reduce all background noise
- touch resident frequently to help them keep in contact with you
- write messages if the resident has good vision

EVERYTHING YOU TOUCH HAS GERMS

Essential Items Needed In Immediate Environment/Room

- Bed/ Linens
- storage space
- chairs
- reading and night light
- call light

Safety Measures

- use good body mechanics
- use clean techniques to prevent spread of germs
- wash hands before and after every tasks
- keep oiled lines (ALL LINENS) away from Uniform
- NEVER put soiled linen on the floor
- prevent clean linen from touching the floor at all times
- **ALWAYS wash hand before and after each linen change**

Additional Responsibilities

- ALWAYS remember to treat the resident's belongings as if you are a visitor
- encourage resident to have their own things
- help safe guard the resident's possessions, after all this is their home, their own room

Ways Micro-Organisms Are Spread

- touches object i.e. Dishes, bed linens, clothing, instruments, resident's belongs
- coughing

Ways Micro-Organisms Are Spread (continued)

- talking
- sneezing
- contaminated food
- airborne transmission = dust particles

Additional Factors That Put A Person At Risk For Infection

Poor nutrition, personal hygiene, hydration, chronic debilitating disease, stress and fatigue

UNIVERSAL PRECAUTIONS

ALWAYS WEAR GLOVES WHEN TOUCHING BLOOD OR ALL BODY FLUIDS (I.E: SECRETIONS COMING OUT OF THE BODY)

ALWAYS WEAR A MASK WHEN PROCEDURE LOSES DROPLETS IN THE AIR (I.E: IF SOMEONE HAS BEEN SNEEZING - COUGHING - SPITTING)

WEAR A GOWN WHEN SPLASHING OF BLOOD OR BODY FLUIDS ARE PRESENT

KNOW YOUR LOCAL POLICY

DEFINITIONS ALWAYS ASKED ON CNA EXAMS

Aphasia = can't put thoughts into words
Cataract = lens thickening, general blurring of vision
Glaucoma = inability to see out of side of eye

REPLACE STRAWS WHEN YOU PUT WATER IN CUPS

Information You Need To Know About Nutrition

FLUIDS

Resident Fluid Intake Needs

- 1500-2000cc per 24 hours
- fresh water
- provide clean cups
- always remind resident to drink during hot weather
- make sure fluids are available
- resident needs 8-10 glasses of water per day

SYMPTOMS OF DEHYDRATION

- signs of being thirsty
- suddenly confused
- more sleepy than usual
- skin easily tinted
- dry eyes and dry mouth
- constipated or watery diarrhea
- dry chapped lips
- urine will be dark brown
- people will have furrows in their tongue

ADDITIONAL INFORMATION

Normal Output 1500cc a day
Know how much each glass holds and accurately record all intake
Measure urine if possible
If incontinent, note number of times they empty

NEVER PUT UP SIDE RAILS UNLESS THE NURSE ORDERS IT

WATER MUST BE WITHIN REACH OF RESIDENT

8 OZ Glass of Water = 240 cc

STATE LAW DURING FEEDING

YOU MUST SIT WITH RESIDENT AT ALL TIMES WHILE WAITING FOR FOOD TO COME TO THE TABLE. HELP THEM TO DRINK FIRST

REASONS FOR HAVING 4 COLORS OF DRINKING GLASSES

Brown Color **Frosted Clear**	=	both brown and frosted indicate regular liquid
Reddish Glasses	=	thin liquid, Fortified Milk for Thin people
Teal Glasses	=	swollen problems - thickened liquids Thickening recipes

Record amount of food that is eaten and report any worsening signs of illness.

NOTE

If there is any difficulty swallowing, or choking, you can clear airway passage with the Heimlich Maneuver

NOTES